150 Practice ECGs:

Interpretation
and
Board Review

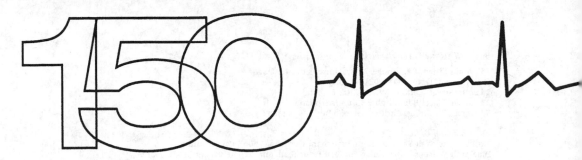

Practice
ECGs:

*Interpretation
and
Board Review*

George J. Taylor, M.D., F.A.C.P.
CLINICAL PROFESSOR OF MEDICINE,
Southern Illinois University School of Medicine,
Prairie Education and Research Cooperative, Springfield, Illinois

**Blackwell
Science**

Blackwell Science Editorial offices:

238 Main Street, Cambridge, Massachusetts 02142, USA
Osney Mead, Oxford OX2 0E1, England
25 John Street, London WC1N 2BL, England
23 Ainslie Place, Edinburgh EH3 6AJ, Scotland
54 University Street, Carlton, Victoria 3053, Australia

Other Editorial Offices:

Arnette Blackwell SA, 224, Boulevard Saint Germain, 75007 Paris, France
Blackwell Wissenschafts-Verlag GmbH Kurfürstendamm 57, 10707 Berlin, Germany
Zehetnergasse 6, A-1140 Vienna, Austria

Distributors:

USA
  Blackwell Science, Inc.
  238 Main Street
  Cambridge, Massachusetts 02142
  (Telephone orders: 800-215-1000 or 617-876-7000
  Fax orders: 617-492-5263)

CANADA
  Copp Clark Professional
  200 Adelaide Street, West, 3rd Floor
  Toronto, Ontario M5H 1W7
  (Telephone orders: 416-597-1616 or 1-800-815-9417;
  Fax: 416-597-1617

AUSTRALIA
  Blackwell Science Pty., Ltd.
  54 University Street
  Carlton, Victoria 3053
  (Telephone orders: 03-9347-0300; Fax orders: 03-9349 3016)

OUTSIDE NORTH AMERICA AND AUSTRALIA
  Blackwell Science, Ltd.
  c/o Marston Book Services, Ltd.
  P.O. Box 269
  Abingdon, Oxon OX14 4YN, England
  (Telephone orders: 44-01235-465500; Fax orders: 44-01235-465555)

Acquisitions: Joy Ferris Denomme
Production: Ellen Samia
Manufacturing: Lisa Flanagan
Cover and Text design: Alwyn R. Velásquez/Lapis Design
Typeset by Achorn Graphics
Printed and bound by Edwards Brothers, Inc.

© 1997 by Blackwell Science, Inc.

Printed in the United States of America
97 98 99   5 4 3 2 1

Library of Congress Cataloging-in-Publication Data

Taylor, George Jesse.
    150 practice ECGs : interpretation and board review / George J. Taylor.
      p.   cm.
    Includes index.
    ISBN 0-86542-233-8 (pbk. : alk. paper)
    1. Electrocardiography—Problems, exercises, etc.
    2. Electrocardiography—Examinations, questions, etc.   I. Title.
    [DNLM: 1. Electrocardiography—problems.   WG 18.2 T241z 1996]
    RC683.5.E5T34   1996
    616.1′207547′076—dc20
    DNLM/DLC
    for Library of Congress   96-38944
                                                                  CIP

To Marilyn

Contents

Preface

Our best teachers are our patients; what we do is called the *practice* of medicine for a good reason. Like most clinicians, I remember little of what I have not used. This brings us to your problem as a student of electrocardiography. You may not get enough practice to become good at it. Most introductory texts do not provide practice. The best way to get experience is to read ECGs from the hospital's daily accumulation, *commit your interpretation to paper,* then look over the shoulder of the experienced person who is reading those ECGs for the record.

Unfortunately, most students and residents do not have that opportunity. Training programs are placing an ever-increasing clinical load on their faculties. One-on-one teaching experiences are hard to program. It is the rare institution that provides *most* of its students and residents headed for primary care practice with an adequate ECG reading experience.

This book is intended as an ECG curriculum that emphasizes practice. My goal is to have you reading ECGs as quickly as possible. The introductory chapters are shorter than those found in the usual beginner's manual, but there is plenty there to get you started. Where you want additional depth, refer to an encyclopedic text in the library. (I especially like the book by T. C. Chou, *Electrocardiography in Clinical Practice*, Grune and Stratton, 1979.)

The practice ECGs include clinical data and questions that are designed to make teaching points. My brief discussion emphasizes daily issues in clinical medicine, as well as material that you may encounter on Board exams (Internal Medicine, Family Practice, Flex, and National Boards). Spend five evenings with these practice ECGs, and you will be far more comfortable than the average house officer with this basic part of the clinical examination.

The high quality of ECG reproduction in this book sets it apart from most other ECG manuals. Credit for this goes to Gordon Grindy and his colleagues at Marquette Electronics, Inc. My thanks to my partner, Wes Moses, who proofread the text and the ECG interpretations. (He is responsible for any

ECG that is misread.) Marsha Strow and Angela Caldieraro, nurse educators at St. John's Hospital, provided many of the rhythm strips. I am especially grateful to Carol Armstrong for the hours she spent at the ECG computer, and to David Lemme, Maria Long, and Brian Burnett, who did the artwork.

My wife, Marilyn, is a patient woman, and I appreciate her forbearance during this writing adventure.

G.J.T.

Normal Intervals

Heart rate   60–99 beats/min
   bradycardia   <60 beats/min
   tachycardia   >100 beats/min
PR   0.12–0.21 sec
   PR prolongation   ≥0.22 sec
QRS   <0.12
QRS axis   −30°–+110°
QTc   QT/√: Normal <0.45 sec

Glossary of Abbreviations

AF   atrial fibrillation
ASD   atrial septal defect
AV   atrioventricular
AVB   atrioventricular block
CHB   complete heart block
ECG   electrocardiogram
HRV   heart rate variability
IRBBB   incomplete right bundle branch block
IVCD   intraventricular conduction delay
LAA   left atrial abnormality
LAD   left axis deviation
LAFB   left anterior fascicular block
LBBB   left bundle branch block
LPFB   left posterior fascicular block
LVII   left ventricular hypertrophy
MAT   multifocal atrial tachycardia
MI   myocardial infarction
MM   millimeter

MV   millivolt
NSR   normal sinus rhythm
NSSTCs   nonspecific ST changes
NSST-TCs   nonspecific ST-T wave changes
NSTWCs   nonspecific T Wave changes
PAC   premature atrial contraction
PAF   paroxysmal atrial fibrillation
PRWP   poor R-wave progression
PSVT   paroxysmal supraventricular tachycardia
PVC   premature ventricular contraction
QTc   corrected QT interval (QTc = QT/square root of RR)
RAA   right atrial abnormality
RAD   right axis deviation
RBBB   right bundle branch block
rT-PA   recombinant tissue plasminogen activator
RVH   right ventricular hypertrophy
SA   sinoatrial
SAN   sinoatrial node
SB   sinus bradycardia
ST   sinus tachycardia (may be confused with the ST segment; the context should clarify this)
SVT   supraventricular tachycardia
VF   ventricular fibrillation
VT   ventricular tachycardia
WPW   Wolff-Parkinson-White syndrome

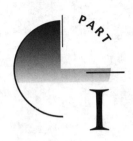

P A R T

I

How to

Interpret

ECGs

Baseline Data

A Protocol for Reading ECGs

The protocol that you should follow when reading ECGs is outlined in Table 1.1. There is nothing new there; it is the method cardiologists have taught generations of students, and it works. After reading ECGs for a living for 20 years, I still use it. With all this practice, I am good at pattern recognition. I glance at an ECG and promptly recognize major abnormalities. As you gain experience, you will develop this ability, and you will be tempted to focus immediately on gross abnormalities that seem to jump out of the page. Resist that temptation! Do what the pros do, and make yourself follow the steps outlined in Table 1.1. Regardless of your ability and experience, if you do not specifically read the rate, rhythm, intervals, and axis, you will miss subtle and important abnormalities. This is one of those areas of clinical medicine where you should not cut corners. Not addressing intervals, for example, would be like omitting the family history from a history and physical exam.

That analogy is a good one. The beauty of the history and physical examination format is that it allows you to collect meaningful data, even when the patient has an illness that you do not understand. Collecting basic data from the ECG serves a similar purpose for the novice.

How to Use This Book

First, read the introductory chapters that explain ECG findings and provide diagnostic criteria for a variety of cardiac conditions. Although important, this exercise will not teach you how to read ECGs. You will take that step when you work through the practice tracings in Part II of this book.

When reading the unknown ECGs in Part II, *write* your interpretation. First, record rate, rhythm, intervals, and QRS axis. Then, analyze QRS and ST-T wave morphologies, and record your impression beginning with ''ECG

Table 1.1 ECG Reading Protocol

The basics	Morphologic changes, interpretation
Rate	Conduction abnormality
Rhythm	Atrial abnormality
Intervals	Ventricular hypertrophy
QRS axis	ST segment–T wave changes
	Patterns of ischemia and infarction

abnormal due to . . ." *If you do not commit yourself on paper, it does not count!* Finally, check your interpretation with mine, which is in the appendix. Read five to ten tracings, or more, before checking answers; there is a kind of rhythm to this activity that you should not interrupt.

Basic clinical data are provided with the ECGs, and I ask questions about management and diagnosis that go beyond the formal ECG report. Reading ECGs is a great time to think (and teach) about heart disease, and I will not miss that opportunity here.

The remainder of this and the next chapter deal with each item on the ECG reading protocol (see Table 1.1). This book is for the near-beginner; most of you have had some introduction to the ECG. I will avoid lengthy description of technical areas such as the origin of lead systems. My goal is to get you through the introductory material as quickly and painlessly as possible, then on to the practice ECGs.

The ECG Is a Voltmeter

That is right. It measures the small amount of voltage generated by depolarization of heart muscle. The vertical, or y axis, on the ECG is *voltage*, with each millimeter (mm) of paper equal to 0.1 millivolt (mV) (Fig 1.1). For practical purposes, we often refer to the amplitude, or height, of an ECG complex in millimeters of paper rather than in millivolts. At the beginning or end of the ECG, you may see a square wave, machine induced, that is 10 mm tall; this is a 1-mV current entered by the machine for calibration. The gain can be changed so that high voltage complexes fit on the paper, or so that low voltage complexes are magnified. Changing the gain is uncommon, but it would be apparent from the calibration marker.

Voltage may have either a negative or a positive value. This is because voltage is a *vector* force with *direction* as well as amplitude. All the rules of vector analysis apply.

Note that the wave of depolarization moves through the heart in three

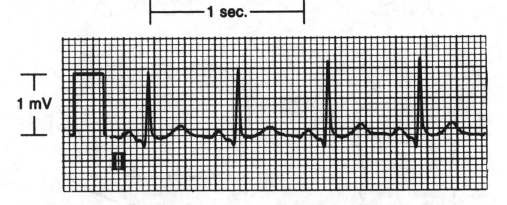

Figure 1.1 The square wave at the beginning is a 1 millivolt calibration marker. At full standard, 10 mm of paper = 1 mV of current. The ECG paper runs at 25 mm/sec. Thus, each mm = 0.04 sec, and each large square (5 mm) = 0.2 sec. The time between two positive deflections, or R waves, is the *RR interval*. If that is one second, the heart rate is 60 beats/min.

dimensions, but that each ECG lead records it in just one dimension, between two poles. Having 12 leads grouped in frontal and horizontal planes allows us to reconstruct electrical events in three dimensions (Fig 1.2). In essence, having 12 leads lets us view the wave of depolarization from multiple angles.

On the ECG, when the wave of depolarization moves toward the positive pole of an individual lead (for example, from the patient's right to the left in lead I) (see Fig 1.2), the deflection is upright, or positive. Downward deflections are negative. The general direction of the wave of depolarization, the orientation of its vector in space, is referred to as the electrical *axis*. This will be discussed at the end of this chapter.

Heart Rate

The ECG records the voltage generated by depolarization of the different regions of the heart *through time*. Following discharge of the sinoatrial (SA) node, the atria are depolarized (the P wave, Fig 1.3). Current then passes through the atrioventricular (AV) node, where there is delay (the PR interval). When the *wave of depolarization* exits the AV node, it passes through the His bundle, then the bundle branches, and on to the ventricles. Discharge of the muscular ventricles produces the QRS complex. This is followed by

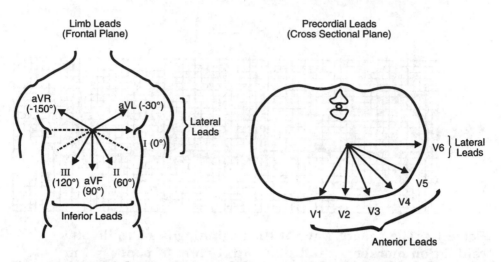

Figure 1.2 Spatial orientation of the 12 ECG leads. Each of the ECG leads functions as a voltmeter and has spatial orientation (as voltage is a vector force). Leads that have an inferior orientation are best at detecting changes from the inferior surface of the heart. Anterior precordial leads are most sensitive in detecting anterior wall changes, and the lateral leads, lateral wall abnormalities.

repolarization of the ventricles (T wave). These events take time. *The ECG paper is moving, and its horizontal, or x, axis is time.*

ECG machines are (arbitrarily) set with a paper speed of 25 mm/sec. At this speed, each millimeter of ECG paper is equal to 1/25, or 0.04 sec (see Fig 1.1). ECG paper is boldly ruled at 5 mm, or 0.2 sec, intervals. And 5 of these large (5 mm) squares equals 1 sec. (All of this is straightforward arithmetic; there is not much rocket science in medicine.)

Using these simple facts, there are two methods for quickly measuring heart rate.

1. Check the distance (that is to say, the time) between two R waves. [The R wave is the dominant and easily identified positive (upright) wave or *deflection* in the QRS complex (see Fig 1.1).] That is the time for one cardiac cycle, or one heartbeat, and it is called the **RR interval.** If the RR interval is 5 large squares, or 1 sec, then one heartbeat takes 1 second, and the rate is 60 beats/min. If the RR interval is 4 squares, or 0.8 sec/beat, then the heart rate is 60 sec/min divided by 0.8 sec/beat, which equals 75 beats/min. Three squares: 60/0.6 = 100 beats/min.

2. A simpler way to do the arithmetic, and the way I determine rate quickly, is to measure the number of large squares between R waves, then divide that into 300: for 2 large squares, rate = 150 beats/min; 3 squares, rate = 100 beats/min; 4 squares, rate = 75/min; 5 squares, rate = 60/min;

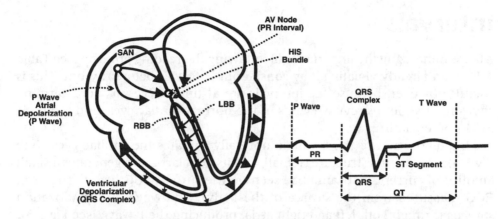

Figure 1.3 Sequence of cardiac activation. The sinoatrial (SA) node, located in the high right atrium, is the cardiac *pacemaker*. It fires at a rate of 60–100 beats/min, and the rate is influenced by both sympathetic and parasympathetic tone. Atrial muscle depolarization produces enough current to cause a deflection, the P wave, on the surface ECG. The wave of depolarization is funneled into the atrioventricular (AV) node, located near the junction of the atrial and ventricular septa. Current is delayed in the AV node, producing the PR interval. This delay allows time for atrial contraction (which completes ventricular filling). Current exits the AV node into the bundle of His, which then divides into the left and right bundle branches. Initial depolarization of the interventricular septum takes place from the left to the right side. Current then moves simultaneously through the left and right bundle branches into the ventricular myocardium, producing the QRS complex. The left ventricle (LV) is much thicker than the right and thus generates more voltage. LV depolarization dominates the QRS complex. The ventricles are then repolarized, producing the T wave on the ECG. Normally, no voltage is apparent between the end of the QRS and the T wave. This ST segment may shift up or down with myocardial ischemia.

6 squares, rate = 50/min; 5.5 squares, rate = between 50 and 60/min. When the rhythm is regular, I select an easily identifiable R wave that falls on, or near, a boldly scored line, then count the number of large squares to the next R wave. It is a crude but fast way to measure rate, but it does not work when the rhythm is grossly irregular. In most cases, it allows you to determine quickly whether the patient has a normal rate, **bradycardia** (less than 60 beats/min), or **tachycardia** (more than 100 beats/min).

Intervals

After emphasizing the importance of following the reading protocol (see Table 1.1), I am already violating it by considering intervals before rhythm. This is useful, however, because the intervals are at times necessary to determine rhythm. First, let us review events of the normal cardiac cycle and the basic ECG nomenclature.

Depolarization of the SA node normally initiates the cardiac cycle (see Fig 1.3). This neural structure is small, and its depolarization generates a small amount of current that cannot be seen on the surface ECG (i.e., the 12-lead ECG measured from the surface of the body). The wave of depolarization spreads through both left and right atria, producing the P wave (see Fig 1.3).

Although the atria and ventricles have a broad area of surface contact, they are effectively insulated from each other. The wave of depolarization from the atrium is funneled through what I think of as a hole in the insulation, but it is actually specialized conducting tissue called the atrioventricular (AV) node. Current moves rapidly along nerves and fairly quickly through heart muscle. But the AV node puts the brakes on the wave of depolarization. This slowing creates a delay between atrial depolarization and ventricular depolarization. A pause in the AV node gives the atria time to contract, providing the final increment of ventricular filling. According to Dr. Starling, that is important; he discovered that greater ventricular volume—or individual muscle fiber length—at the beginning of ventricular contraction produces stronger contraction.

PR Interval

The interval that includes a measure of the AV node conduction delay is the PR interval (see Fig 1.3). It is often easier to identify the beginning of the P wave than its end, and by convention, this interval is measured from the start of the P wave. The interval thus includes the time of atrial depolarization, the P wave itself, and the delay during AV node conduction (roughly the time from the end of the P wave until the beginning of the QRS complex). However, when the PR interval is prolonged, it is usually a result of delayed AV node conduction; I know of no condition that lengthens the P wave enough to cause prolongation of the PR interval.

A common question is *which ECG lead to use* for measuring the PR or other intervals. What you are trying to measure with the PR interval is the time from initiation of atrial depolarization until the beginning of ventricular depolarization. There are slight variations in the sensitivities of particular ECG leads for recording the onset of the P wave, and which lead is most sensitive will vary from patient to patient. It makes sense to use the lead that records atrial depolarization earliest and ventricular depolarization earliest.

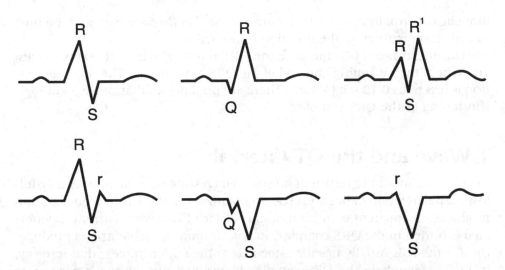

Figure 1.4 QRS nomenclature. Any positive deflection is an R wave. An initial negative deflection is a Q wave. A negative deflection following an R wave is an S wave. Small, low-voltage deflections may be designated with lowercase letters. When there are two R waves separated by an S wave, the second may be referred to as R′ (R-prime).

Do you get the feeling that these are rough measurements, despite the fact that we are dealing with milliseconds and microvolts? The truth is that they are, and that the surface ECG is a crude tool. As a practical matter, measure intervals from a lead where the onset of the waves—P and QRS—is well defined, and where the interval seems longest. This general rule applies to the measurement of all intervals.

The normal PR interval ranges from 0.12 to 0.22 sec (see page xi). First-degree atrioventricular block (1°AV block) is defined as a PR interval of 0.22 sec or more.

QRS Duration

Ventricular depolarization produces the QRS complex, the largest deflection on the ECG (see Fig 1.3). As a rule, the voltage generated is proportional to the amount of muscle depolarized, and the ventricles contain the bulk of cardiac muscle. QRS nomenclature may seem confusing at first, but it follows quite simple conventions (Fig 1.4).

The *QRS duration*, or interval, is a measure of the time it takes to depolarize the two ventricles. Look again at Figure 1.3. Current exits the AV node and the His bundle and moves *simultaneously* through the infranodal bundle branches. Normally, the ventricles are activated *at the same time*, and the time of activation is roughly the duration of the QRS.

On the surface ECG, measure the QRS duration where it seems longest and where the beginning and end of the QRS are obvious. The normal duration is less than 0.12 sec (3 mm). There are no illnesses that cause pathologic shortening of the QRS complex.

T Wave and the QT Interval

Repolarization, or the return of muscle to its resting state, spontaneously follows depolarization in heart muscle. Repolarization of the thin-walled atrium produces no apparent deflection on the surface ECG; what current is generated is buried in the QRS complex. Repolarization of the ventricles produces the *T wave*. This usually has the same axis as the QRS complex; that is to say, in ECG leads where the QRS complex is positive, the T wave is positive as well.

Think back to physiology and recall the shape of the action potential of isolated nerve or muscle cells. Repolarization, or the return of the cell membrane to resting potential after depolarization, is a brief event, a sharp downward deflection. However, the repolarization wave on the surface ECG is broad. That is because the T wave reflects repolarization of the large population of cardiac cells, some of which repolarize early and others much later. The T wave looks like a bell-shaped curve; in some ways it is, with the average cell repolarizing at the peak of the T wave. A broader T wave would indicate temporal dispersion of repolarization (technospeak from electrophysiologists), or greater heterogeneity of the repolarization process among cardiac muscle cells so that it takes longer (*temporal dispersion* means *takes longer*). Remember that a *broader* wave just means that time, measured along the x axis of the ECG, is longer.

All this is clinically important, because increased heterogeneity of repolarization underlies the pathogenesis of serious cardiac arrhythmias. A long *QT interval* (a measure of the duration of repolarization) may identify the patient at risk for ventricular arrhythmias and sudden death.

The QT interval is measured from the *beginning* of the QRS complex to the end of the T wave (see Fig 1.3). Why measure from the beginning of the QRS, apart from convention? It is probably because the beginning of the QRS often is easier to identify than the end, and the QRS complex is short relative to the duration of the QT interval. Measure the QT interval using the lead where it seems longest.

The normal duration of the QT interval varies with heart rate. The corrected QT (QTc) is calculated using Dr. Bazett's formula:

$$QTc = QT\sqrt{RR \text{ interval}}$$

The RR interval, or the duration of one cardiac cycle, is a measure of heart rate. Therefore, when the heart rate is 60 beats/min, and the RR interval is 1 sec, the QTc equals the QT (measured). When the heart rate is greater than 60 beats/min and the RR interval is less than 1 sec, the QTc will be greater than the measured QT. Most ECG manuals provide tables that give the top-normal QT (measured) for a given heart rate, and these tables are based on Bazett's formula with top normal QTc < 0.45 sec.

There is a quick and easy method for determining whether the QT interval is normal, and it is the method I use when plowing through a stack of ECGs. If the measured QT is less than half the RR interval, then it is probably normal. If it is clearly longer, then it is probably abnormal. Using this short-cut, my ECG interpretation usually reads QT normal for the rate or QT prolonged for the rate. In borderline situations, and when the QT is long, I calculate the QTc (or use the table on page xi). I find that the ECG computer is occasionally inaccurate with its automatic measurement of the QT interval. Particularly with rapid heart rates, there is a tendency to overdiagnose QT prolongation, even with careful measurement.

The T wave may contain a second hump, or even a separate wave, which is called the U wave, and this is a part of the ventricular repolarization process. It may be a normal finding. There is general agreement that it should be considered a part of the T wave when thinking of QT, or QTU, prolongation. Hypokalemia, especially in combination with hypomagnesemia, causes an increase in U wave amplitude and prolongation of the QTU interval.

QT interval prolongation is important. You will miss it unless you look for it on every ECG you read. One place you will see it is on Board exams. Conditions and drugs that prolong the QT interval are summarized in Table 1.2.

Table 1.2 Conditions and Drugs Affecting Intervals and Morphologies

INTERVAL	CONDITION (CARDIAC AND NONCARDIAC)	DRUGS/METABOLIC ABNORMALITY
PR	1° AV block	Digoxin, beta adrenergic blockers, calcium blockers, intravenous adenosine
QRS	Ventricular conduction abnormalities, including bundle branch block; pre-excitation	Quinidine, flecainide, propafenone and other antiarrhythmics; extreme hyperkalemia
QT/QTU	Myocardial ischemia, hypothermia, intracranial bleeding, long QT syndrome	Quinidine, procainamide, disopyramide, sotalol, amiodarone, phenothiazine and phenothiazine derivatives, erythromycin; hypokalemia, hypomagnesemia, hypocalcemia

Table 1.2 Conditions and Drugs Affecting Intervals and Morphologies (continued)

	DRUGS	METABOLIC CONDITIONS
Interval Prolongation		
QRS Morphology		
Q waves	None	None
ST Segment		
Depression	Digitalis	None
Elevation	None	None
T Waves		
Increased amplitude	None	Hyperkalemia
Inversion	None	None
U Waves	None	Hypokalemia

Rhythm

My purpose is to help the student read through a stack of ECGs in the heart station (and look good to the attending). I will review *selected rhythms* common in this setting, but I will not attempt a comprehensive discussion of the rhythm abnormalities that you will encounter in telemetry units.

Sinus Rhythm and Sinus Arrhythmia

Normal Sinus Rhythm

Normal sinus rhythm (NSR) is a regular rhythm between 60 and 100 beats/min, with a P wave before each QRS complex and a QRS after each P wave. A faster rate defines *tachycardia* and a slower rate, *bradycardia*. The term *sinus* indicates that the rhythm originates in the SA node, that there is atrial depolarization (a P wave before each QRS), and that atrial contraction precedes ventricular contraction.

Sinus Tachycardia

When you are excited, or when you walk up stairs and are short-winded and your pulse is 120 beats/min, you probably have *sinus tachycardia*. It is benign rhythm, right? Actually, that depends on the clinical setting. It is a normal response of healthy people to exercise. But sinus tachycardia in a patient who is at rest and pain free the day after a myocardial infarction (MI) may indicate a large MI with heart failure. Although the rhythm does not require specific treatment, it makes me fearful for the patient's survival, because it indicates poor left ventricular function. In patients with other kinds of heart disease, sinus tachycardia may also indicate decompensation. There are noncardiac illnesses that may cause sinus tachycardia, such as thyrotoxicosis, anemia, and fever. It may also be caused by drugs, such as thyroid hormone, catecholamines, caffeine, and amphetamines.

Sinus Bradycardia

Sinus bradycardia (SB) is a common finding. In the absence of conduction abnormalities, when all the intervals are normal, bradycardia at rest is usually a normal variant. It may be an indicator of good cardiovascular fitness, and it is common in trained athletes. It can be a drug effect (e.g., digitalis, beta adrenergic blockers, or calcium channel blockers). A variety of illnesses can cause sinus slowing, including the sick sinus syndrome, hypothyroidism, and sleep apnea (and other conditions that cause hypoxemia). Vasovagal attacks may cause profound sinus bradycardia, sinus pauses, and syncope, but these are transient and usually are not observed on 12-lead ECGs.

Sinus Arrhythmia

Sinus arrhythmia usually indicates good cardiovascular health. During the respiratory cycle, the vagus nerve is intermittently activated, producing a beat-to-beat variation in heart rate. On the 12-lead ECG (which is a relatively short rhythm strip), this is seen as a variable RR interval. When pronounced, it may affect your quick and easy calculation of heart rate using the technique just described. Be aware of this, but do not worry as long as the rate is within the normal limits.

Sinus arrhythmia may disappear when the heart is sick, as in the case of heart failure. The autonomic nervous system compensates for low cardiac output by activating the sympathetic nervous system and suppressing the parasympathetic nervous system. Resting heart rate increases. Additionally, the vagus nerve is not activated during the respiratory cycle, and there is little if any variation in RR intervals. The rhythm becomes perceptibly more regular.

Measurement of **heart rate variability (HRV)** has emerged as a noninvasive test for increased risk of ventricular arrhythmias. You might think of vagal activity as being protective against dangerous ventricular arrhythmias, although in reality, vagal activity may be more an indicator of good left ventricular function (and therefore of a low risk of arrhythmias) than a protector.

Low HRV (reduced vagal tone) indicates high risk, and increased HRV (more sinus arrhythmia, higher vagal tone) means lower risk. HRV may be measured by calculating the mean and standard deviation of a large number of RR intervals; the standard deviation serves as a measure of the variability. Electrophysiologists have also used *power spectral analysis* of RR intervals (sounds like a black box to me). This mathematical approach allows separation of HRV into vagal and sympathetic components.

In addition to heart disease, *autonomic dysfunction* caused by a variety of neurologic conditions may also affect HRV, but without increasing the risk of ventricular arrhythmias. These include alcoholism, diabetic and uremic neuropathy, and the Guillain-Barré syndrome. Dysfunction of medullary centers that control autonomic function may also reduce HRV (e.g., cerebral hypoxia and/or brain death).

Heart Block

Block can be a confusing term in cardiovascular medicine. Blocked arteries, blocked valves, and blocked nerve conduction are different illnesses, but they may be confused by patients (and medical students). The term *heart block* usually refers to interruption of nerve conduction. It is an electrical problem, not one of fuel lines or valves (although these conditions often coexist).

Nerve conduction can be interrupted, or blocked, at any level of the cardiac nervous system (see Fig 1.3). Block is uncommon within the SA node or in the body of the atrium. But it is quite common in the AV node and in the nerves below the AV node (see Fig 1.3). These infranodal nerves include the His bundle, the bundle branches and their major divisions, and the small terminal Purkinje fibers. The infranodal nerves may be referred to as the *His-Purkinje system*.

Blocked conduction may alter intervals and may cause bradycardia. When block is complete, there is no transmission to structures distal to the block, but the heart rarely stops. Instead, an *auxiliary* pacemaker just below the level of block takes over. The intrinsic rate of the takeover pacemaker is progressively slower the farther it is from the SA node. Control of heart rate reminds me of the children's game King of the Mountain. Pacers highest on the mountain, nearest the SA node, get the first chance to rule. When they fail, those just below take over. As you go lower down the mountain, the pacers are slower.

For example, when complete block occurs in the AV node, a pacemaker in the His bundle, just below the AV node, takes over with an intrinsic rate of 30 to 45 beats/min. It would be hard to exercise with a heart rate that slow, but with that rate, syncope is uncommon. If complete block occurs farther down, within the septum and beyond the division of the two bundle

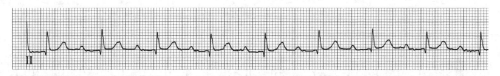

Figure 1.5 First-degree AV block. The PR interval is longer than 0.22 sec, and it does not vary.

branches (see Fig 1.3), the takeover pacemaker is in the body of the ventricles. These deeper pacers have a much slower intrinsic rate, occasionally as slow as 10 to 20 beats/min. In this case, syncope and even sudden death are more likely than in the case of a takeover pacemaker higher in the conduction system.

In addition to a slower intrinsic rate, takeover pacemakers from within the body of the ventricle are less responsive to the autonomic nervous system. A pacemaker in the AV node, or just below it, may respond to catecholamines with an increase in rate. But deeper, ventricular pacemakers exhibit little change in rate with sympathetic stimulation.

From this outline of general principles, you begin to see that the level of block determines prognosis, and identification of this level is critical. Now we turn to specific ECG findings and clinical situations.

First-Degree AV Block

First-degree AV block is defined as a PR interval of 0.22 sec or more, and without variation (Fig 1.5). It is caused by a delay in conduction in the AV node. Increased vagal tone, hyperkalemia, digitalis, calcium blockers (particularly diltiazem and verapamil), and beta adrenergic blockers all may slow AV node conduction. It is common in elderly patients, who may have primary degeneration of the AV node in the absence of ischemic heart disease. In other patients, ischemia may injure the AV node and either delay or block conduction. The right coronary artery usually supplies the AV node as well as the inferior wall of the heart. AV nodal block is relatively common with inferior myocardial infarction (which may also be complicated by increased vagal tone).

Second-Degree Heart Block, Mobitz I (Wenckebach) and II

With second-degree AV block, some beats pass through the AV node to the ventricles, but others do not. This follows a pattern: when every other P wave captures the ventricle (producing a QRS complex), the patient is said to have

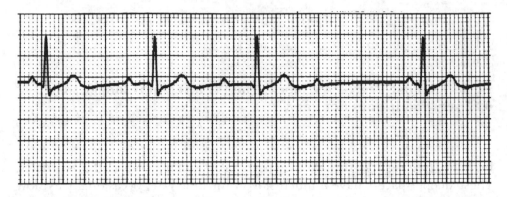

Figure 1.6 Second-degree AV block, Mobitz type I (or Wenckebach). The level of block is the AV node. There is progressive lengthening of the PR interval until the P wave is not conducted. After the dropped beat, the PR interval is short (the AV node has had time to recuperate). An additional feature, not mentioned in the text, is progressive shortening of the RR interval before the dropped beat. Note that the QRS complex is narrow; more evidence that the level of block is the AV node.

2:1 block. When every third P wave is conducted through the AV node, it is 3:1 block; and when 2 of 3 P waves are conducted, it is 3:2 block.

Second-degree heart block is further classified into two types, **Mobitz I and II.** This is a source of confusion. (I find it easier to remember without the Mobitz designations, instead thinking anatomically of where in the conduction system block occurs.)

Mobitz I block usually occurs *within the AV node.* (We have to use qualifiers like *usually*; in the case of Mobitz I block, the exceptions are rare.) Injury to the node causes it to tire with each succeeding beat until it is so tired that a P wave is completely blocked. On the ECG, we observe progressive prolongation of the PR interval until there is a P wave that is blocked and not followed by a QRS (Fig 1.6). This is also called the **Wenckebach phenomenon.** Notice that the PR interval of the beat following the blocked beat, or pause, is shorter. It seems that the AV node recuperates during the pause.

Mobitz I block occurs at the level of the AV node, and the conduction system below the node may be normal. With normal intraventricular conduction, the QRS duration is normal. In fact, normal QRS duration excludes block below the AV node. On the other hand, a wide QRS does not define block as infranodal. It is possible for a patient with a preexisting intraventricular conduction abnormality (and wide QRS) to develop AV nodal disease.

Recognition of Mobitz I or Wenckebach AV block   Think of Mobitz I or Wenckebach when you see group beating (groups of QRS complexes regularly

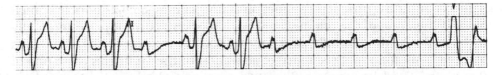

Figure 1.7 Second-degree AV block, Mobitz type II. The patient initially drops a single beat, and this dropped beat is an example of Mobitz II block. He then goes into complete heart block. The last beat is a ventricular escape beat. The PR interval of conducted beats is fixed; there is no evidence of the Wenckebach phenomenon. In addition, the QRS complex is wide; the 12-lead ECG showed bifascicular block (Chapter 2). A wide QRS, indicating abnormal intraventricular conduction, is invariably seen in patients with infranodal heart block.

separated by pauses). Look for progressive prolongation of the PR, then a P wave not followed by a QRS, and then a shorter PR interval following the blocked beat.

Mobitz II block, another form of second-degree block, is caused by block *below the AV node.* The AV node may be healthy. This form of block does not cause progressive prolongation of the PR interval in the beats preceding the blocked beat (Fig 1.7). Because the infranodal conduction system is diseased, the QRS is wide (there is an intraventricular conduction abnormality). A narrow QRS excludes infranodal heart block. Mobitz II block often precedes symptomatic, complete heart block (see Fig 1.7) and may be an indicator for pacemaker implantation.

2:1 AV Block—Is It Mobitz I or II?

Mobitz I second-degree AV block can be severe enough that every other beat is blocked (i.e., 2:1 AV block). This would eliminate progressive lengthening of the PR interval as a diagnostic marker. In fact, 2:1 AV block is a common rhythm with digitalis toxicity; it is of the Mobitz I variety, as the level of block is the AV node. How do you know whether 2:1 block is Mobitz I or Mobitz II? One way is to get a long rhythm strip: with Mobitz I block, there may be brief sections where block will be less severe, with 3:2 or 4:3 conduction and typical PR interval findings.

Another way to tell is to focus on the QRS duration. I am repeating this because it is important. When block occurs at the level of the AV node, the infranodal conduction system usually is healthy, the ventricles are activated in the normal sequence (that is, simultaneously), and the QRS duration is normal. When block occurs below the AV node (i.e., Mobitz II block), the patient has intraventricular conduction abnormalities such as bundle branch block. When one of the bundle branches is blocked, current passes normally through the healthy bundle, and later works its way over to the side that is blocked. This abnormal sequence of activation of the ventricles, with one of them stimulated late, causes the QRS duration to be longer. (More about bundle branch block in the next chapter.)

As noted above, it is possible for an elderly person to have infranodal disease with bundle branch block, plus a sick AV node and Mobitz I block. This occasionally needs sorting out in the electrophysiology lab when there is uncertainty about a need for pacemaker therapy.

Third-Degree, Complete Heart Block

Complete AV nodal block is just that; nothing gets through the AV node. There are P waves and QRS complexes, but they are unrelated; this may be called **AV dissociation** (Fig 1.8). The term may be used when a P wave is not followed by a QRS, so that the atria and ventricles operate independently. Complete heart block is just one of the conditions where this occurs, and you will encounter other examples in Chapter 2.

How do you know whether block occurs within the AV node itself, or in the infranodal conduction system? The issues are those discussed above with 2:1 AV block. When block is at the level of the AV node, the takeover pacemaker is just below the node, within the His bundle and before the division into the bundle branches (see Fig 1.3). The sequence of ventricular activation is therefore normal, and the QRS duration is normal (unless there is coexisting bundle branch block). Furthermore, the takeover pacemaker is relatively high in the conduction system and has an intrinsic rate ranging from 35 to 45 beats/min. The rate would probably increase with catecholamine infusion or administration of atropine. When complete block develops in the infranodal conduction system, the takeover pacer is in the body of the ventricle, the QRS is wide, and the rate is slow (this is called an **idioventricular rhythm** or pacemaker). It probably will not respond to atropine or catecholamines.

Infranodal complete heart block is common among elderly patients, often causing syncope. It may also present as increased fatigue or heart failure. In this age group, the usual cause is fibrotic degeneration of the infranodal nerves (frayed wires). When it occurs in younger people, consider ischemic injury of these nerves; this usually occurs in a setting of large, anterior myocardial infarction. Regardless of etiology or the age of the patient, infranodal complete heart block is an indication for pacemaker therapy.

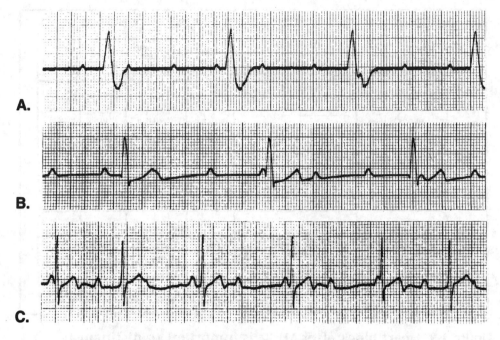

Figure 1.8 Three patients with complete heart block. The atria are being discharged at a regular rate (P waves), and the ventricles at a regular rate (QRS complexes). The two rhythms appear unrelated; there is _AV dissociation_. You may be tempted to say that P waves coming before QRS complexes could be conducted, but these do not alter the regularity of the ventricular escape rhythm.

Patients A and B have wide QRS complexes and slow ventricular rates; they probably have block below the AV node, and the takeover pacemakers are ventricular in origin. Patient C has a more rapid escape rate (55 beats/min), and the QRS complex is narrow; the level of block is probably the AV node.

Heart Block with Acute Myocardial Infarction

Heart block is a common complication of inferior MI, and it is infrequent with anterior MI (Fig 1.9). It helps to remember how the location of block determines the severity of the arrhythmia and prognosis. Heart block with _inferior MI_ probably has dual causation. First, patients with inferior MI have high vagal tone, possibly related to the Bezold-Jarisch reflex. Second, there may be ischemia of the AV node, as the AV node is supplied by the same artery that feeds the inferior wall. You may expect the usual features of AV nodal block: PR interval prolongation and Mobitz I patterns are common, the

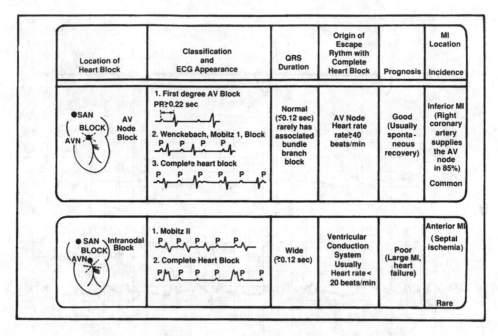

Location of Heart Block	Classification and ECG Appearance	QRS Duration	Origin of Escape Rythm with Complete Heart Block	Prognosis	MI Location Incidence
●SAN BLOCK AVN AV Node Block	1. First degree AV Block PR≥0.22 sec 2. Wenckebach, Mobitz 1, Block P P P P 3. Complete heart block P P P P P P	Normal (≤0.12 sec) rarely has associated bundle branch block	AV Node Heart rate rate≥40 beats/min	Good (Usually sponta- neous recovery)	Inferior MI (Right coronary artery supplies the AV node in 85%) Common
● SAN BLOCK AVN Infranodal Block	1. Mobitz II P P P P P 2. Complete Heart Block PM P P P MP P	Wide (≥0.12 sec)	Ventricular Conduction System Usually Heart rate < 20 beats/min	Poor (Large MI, heart failure)	Anterior MI (Septal ischemia) Rare

Figure 1.9 Heart block after MI. It is important to distinguish between block at the level of the AV node and block below the AV node. The takeover pacemaker with AV nodal block has an adequate intrinsic rate and responds to atropine. Deep ventricular pacemakers that take over after infranodal block are less responsive and are too slow.

QRS is narrow, and the takeover pacer is fairly rapid if block is complete. In addition, the AV node usually has collateral blood flow from other arteries, so permanent injury is uncommon and recovery of normal conduction is the rule. Permanent pacemaker therapy is rarely needed, although temporary pacing is indicated for symptomatic bradycardia. The heart rate usually responds to atropine therapy.

Anterior MI may injure the interventricular septum below the AV node, so the pattern of heart block is infranodal: Mobitz II block is the rule, the QRS is wide, and, when block is complete, the escape rhythm is slow. An anterior infarction large enough to cause infranodal block is usually huge, spontaneous recovery from the heart block is rare, and the prognosis is terrible. These patients need pacemakers, but despite pacing, they do poorly because of the degree of LV injury.

Atrial Arrhythmias

These arrhythmias may be chronic or acute. They are common, and you will see them almost daily when reading routine ECGs.

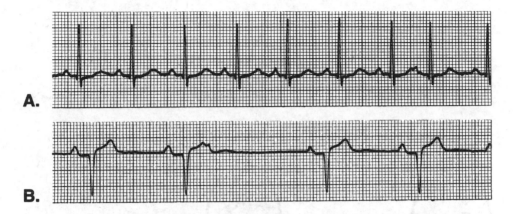

Figure 1.10　Two patients with premature atrial contractions (PAC's). A: An ectopic P wave is seen before the premature QRS. B: Blocked PAC, causing a pause. The ectopic P wave is seen as a distortion of the preceding T wave. This is a common cause of pauses. In most cases, the ectopic P wave is harder to see; look for subtle changes in the preceding T wave.

Premature Atrial Contractions

Premature atrial contractions (PAC's), also called PAB's (beats) or APB's, are usually easy to recognize. The premature beat has a narrow QRS, and the QRS looks like those of normal sinus beats. There may be a misshapen, ectopic P wave before it (Fig 1.10).

A **blocked PAC** may be the cause of a pause on the ECG or rhythm strip, a pause that may be felt by the patient (see Fig 1.10). This happens when the PAC is early enough that the AV node is refractory and will not conduct it. The P wave that is blocked may be buried in the T wave of the preceding complex, making it hard to see. Look for subtle alteration in the T wave just before the pause. This is a favorite Board question.

PAC's are common in young, healthy people and do not indicate heart disease.

Paroxysmal Supraventricular Tachycardia

Paroxysmal supraventricular tachycardia (PSVT) is a rapid, regular rhythm with a rate of 120 to 200 beats/min. Most cases are caused by reentry within the AV node.

Reentry　Before going further with PSVT, we need to discuss **reentry** as a mechanism of premature beats and tachyarrhythmias. The concept is one that

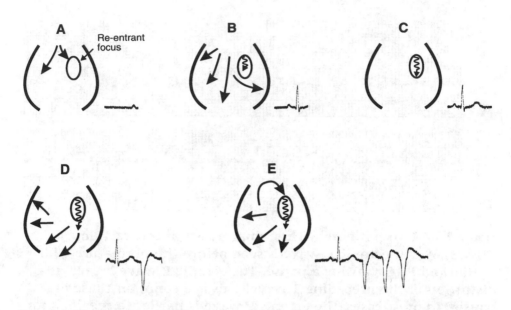

Figure 1.11 Reentry. Follow the sequence of events. A: The wave of depolarization comes from above (the atrium in the case of atrial arrhythmias, the ventricle in this case of ventricular reentry). B: As current moves through the myocardium, it also enters the reentrant focus, a region that is insulated from the surrounding tissue. C: Depolarization of the surrounding myocardium happens quickly, but conduction through the reentrant focus is slow. D: By the time current exits the reentrant focus, the surrounding tissue has been repolarized and is *vulnerable*. That is to say, it can be stimulated. This produces the *ectopic beat*. E: If the timing is perfect, current from the ectopic beat reenters the protected focus, travels through it, and again finds the surrounding tissue vulnerable when it exits. A circuit is established and the result is repetitive ectopic beats.

Characteristics of the reentrant focus that make this possible: 1) Insulation from surrounding tissue, 2) unidirectional conduction, and 3) slow conduction.

is often misunderstood, but is actually quite simple (Fig 1.11). The reentrant focus is a region that is protected, or insulated, from surrounding tissue. Current enters one end of the focus, and it exits the other (conduction is unidirectional). Within the focus, conduction is much slower than conduction through the surrounding tissue. By the time current exits the focus, the surrounding tissue has depolarized and has had time to repolarize as well. Thus, the current exiting the focus finds the surrounding tissue vulnerable, ready

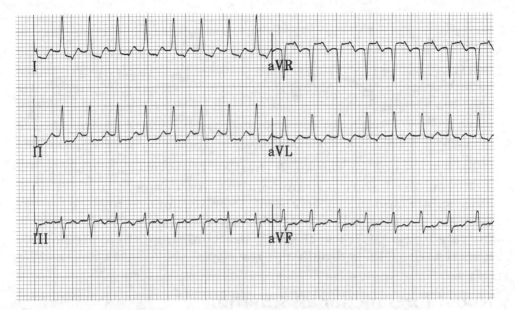

Figure 1.12 Paroxysmal supraventricular tachycardia (PSVT), a recording of limb leads. The rate is 200 beats/min. The T waves appear distorted, and these distortions may be the ectopic P waves. This episode lasted 45 min, plenty of time to get an ECG.

to be stimulated, and that is just what happens: a premature beat is generated. This seems to be the mechanism of many atrial and ventricular premature beats. A reentrant focus in the atrium would cause a PAC, and a focus in the body of the ventricle, a premature ventricular contraction (PVC).

If the timing is perfect, the premature beat may slip back into the entrance of the reentrant focus, leading to another or even to a series of ectopic beats. A circuit is created (see Fig 1.11).

Now back to PSVT. In most cases, the reentrant focus is near or within the body of the AV node. Current exiting the reentrant focus is coming from the AV node and passes normally through the His bundle. The QRS complex is therefore narrow (unless there is coexisting bundle branch block). PSVT is thus a **narrow complex tachycardia** (Fig 1.12).

PSVT is a common and occasionally recurrent arrhythmia in otherwise healthy young people. It is not dangerous or fatal, but it can be bothersome, causing palpitations, dizziness, and near-syncope. It is uncommon for patients to lose consciousness. When symptoms are frequent or are not easily controlled by medical therapy, *ablation of the reentrant focus* within the AV node is possible using catheter techniques. This is a cure (we do not do much of that in cardiology), and many patients prefer this to life-long drug therapy.

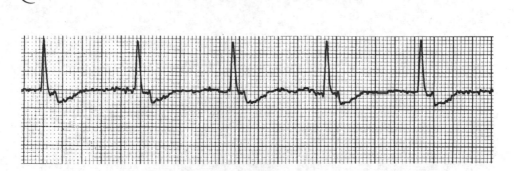

Figure 1.13 Nodal (or *junctional*) rhythm. The retrograde P wave distorting the T wave is prominent in this example. Usually it is more subtle, and it may be absent. Even without retrograde P waves, the diagnosis of junctional rhythm may be made when the rate is regular, is less than 100 beats/min, and there are no P waves. The QRS is usually narrow.

Nodal (or Junctional) Rhythm

This is recognized by the absence of P waves before the QRS, and the rhythm is regular. Although tachycardia (rate ≥ 100) is possible, the heart rate usually is within the normal range. As stimulation of the ventricle comes from the AV node, the QRS is narrow. There may be retrograde activation of the atria, and inverted *(retrograde)* P waves may be seen distorting the T waves (Fig 1.13).

Atrial Fibrillation

It is a rare day that I read ECGs and fail to see a few cases of atrial fibrillation (AF). A grossly irregular rhythm without P waves indicates the diagnosis (Fig 1.14). The rate is usually less than 120, as most patients with chronic AF have already had the ventricular rate, or *response*, controlled with drugs that slow AV nodal conduction (e.g., digoxin, beta adrenergic blockers, or the calcium blockers, verapamil and diltiazem). Students often are fooled by more rapid rates in which the irregular irregularities may be subtle (see Fig 1.14). Atrial fibrillation is not an example of AV dissociation. The atria may be beating (or fibrillating) at rates as high as 600 beats/min, but the ventricle is stimulated (captured) by atrial beats that traverse the AV node. Fibrillation waves may be low voltage and invisible, but often they are coarse enough to distort the baseline (see Fig 1.14).

Atrial Flutter

Atrial flutter is a regular rhythm. The atrial rate is typically 300 beats/min. A patient with a ventricular rate of 150/min has 2:1 AV block; 3:1 AV block

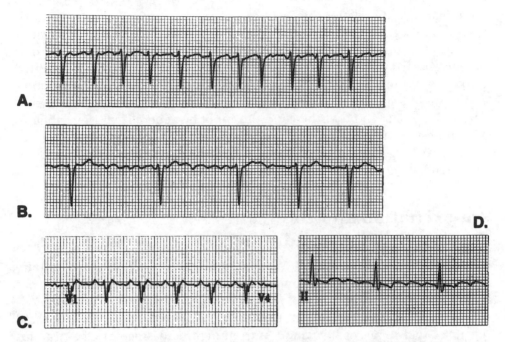

Figure 1.14 Four patients with supraventricular tachyarrhythmia. A: Atrial fibrillation (AF) with rapid ventricular response; at higher rates, the variation in the RR interval seen with AF may be subtle. B: AF with a controlled ventricular response; with drug therapy to slow AV node conduction, the ventricular rate is kept between 80 and 100/min. In this case, you can see the fibrillation waves as coarse undulation in the baseline. C: Atrial flutter with 2:1 block; note the sawtooth pattern in the baseline. D: Atrial flutter with 4:1 block; the flutter waves are more obvious.

produces a ventricular rate of 100/min. Flutter waves with a sawtooth appearance are usually apparent in at least one ECG lead (see Fig 1.14). When you see a regular rate at 150/min on a telemetry rhythm strip, think of atrial flutter and order a 12-lead ECG to look for flutter waves.

At times, flutter waves (which are P waves) cannot be seen on the surface ECG, and it is not possible to tell whether the patient has atrial flutter or PSVT, because both are narrow QRS complex tachyarrhythmias that may have a ventricular rate around 150 beats/min. Placing an ECG lead closer to the heart, using an esophageal or right atrial electrode, allows detection of P waves. In fact, the P waves look huge when measured from the right atrium. With PSVT, there is one P wave with each QRS, and with flutter there are two for each QRS (2:1 block).

Atrial flutter, like atrial fibrillation, is not an example of AV dissociation.

There is a definite relationship between atria and ventricles, with P waves intermittently getting through the AV node and stimulating the ventricles.

New atrial flutter in an elderly, bedridden patient with minimal symptoms may be an early sign of pulmonary embolus. One of my teachers suggested thinking of flutter as a rhythm originating in the right atrium, and atrial fibrillation as a left atrial arrhythmia. I realize that this is simplistic, that there is plenty of overlap, and that the concept cannot be generalized. Nevertheless, it is interesting how often flutter complicates pulmonary problems such as obstructive lung disease or pulmonary embolus. Atrial fibrillation, on the other hand, is a common complication of hypertension (a left-sided problem).

Pre-excitation and the Wolff-Parkinson-White Syndrome

The Wolff-Parkinson-White (WPW) syndrome gives us another opportunity to think about reentry. It is a common problem, and it is a favorite of Board examiners.

Normally, there is a layer of connective tissue separating the atria and ventricles that serves as insulation, preventing free passage of electrical impulses between the upper and lower chambers (Fig 1.15). The AV node is the normal passage through this layer of insulation. Pre-excitation of the ventricle occurs because of an *additional defect* in the insulation between atria and

---

Figure 1.15 Pre-excitation (or the Wolff-Parkinson-White syndrome). This cartoon illustrates the changes caused by a bypass tract between the atria and ventricles. The tract is located on the LV side and near the mitral valve in this particular patient, but bypass tracts may be located at any site where atria and ventricles come into contact. Simultaneous activation of the ventricles via the bypass tract and the AV node produces a fusion beat. Conduction through the bypass tract is faster than through the AV node. Early activation of the ventricle produces the delta wave and makes the PR interval appear short.

A reentrant circuit can develop between the bypass tract and the AV node, resulting in supraventricular tachycardia. There are two possibilities. A: The reentrant circuit moves antegrade through the AV node, retrograde through the bypass tract. The sequence of ventricular activation is therefore normal, and the QRS is narrow. B: The reentrant circuit is directed retrograde through the AV node and antegrade through the bypass tract. Because activation of the ventricles originates from the lateral wall of the LV, the QRS complex is wide.

Preexcitation of the left ventricle through a bypass tract

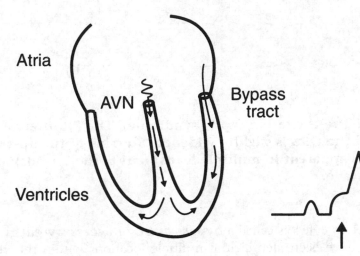

Atria

AVN

Bypass tract

Ventricles

delta wave

Two patterns of supraventricular tachycardia

A.

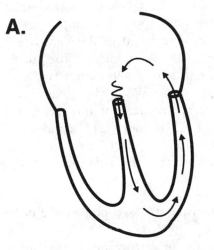

Narrow QRS complex tachycardia

B.

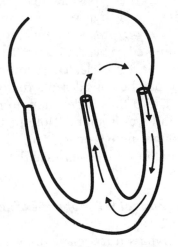

Wide QRS complex tachycardia

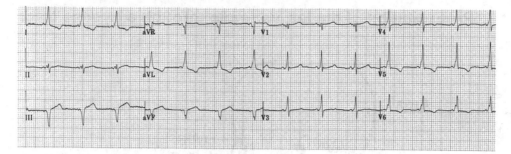

Figure 1.16 Pre-excitation (WPW syndrome). The PR interval is short, and the QRS is slightly widened. Slurring of the upstroke of the QRS is apparent in multiple leads (I, aVL, the V leads); this is the *delta* wave.

ventricles. This defect is called a **bypass tract,** or **accessory pathway.** Bypass tracts have been identified at multiple locations within this region of surface contact between atria and ventricles. WPW refers to the most common of these bypass tract locations, and *pre-excitation* is the more generic term for any syndrome involving a bypass tract between atria and ventricles (WPW is thus a subset of pre-excitation).

As the wave of depolarization passes through the atria, it leaks through the bypass tract as well as into the AV node (see Fig 1.15). Conduction through the bypass tract is usually faster than AV nodal conduction. As current exits the bypass tract, it stimulates ventricular depolarization; the ventricle is *pre-excited,* a catchy way of saying that a segment of the ventricle is stimulated early. An instant later, current exits the AV node and also stimulates the ventricle. The ventricular complex thus originates from two sites and may be considered a **fusion beat.**

The QRS is wider than normal and starts earlier after the P wave, so the PR interval is short. (Note that this does not reflect more rapid conduction through the AV node.) The initial, slurred portion of the QRS caused by pre-excitation of the ventricle through the bypass tract is the *delta wave* (see Fig 1.15).

Diagnosis of WPW or pre-excitation PR interval <0.12 sec, plus a delta wave (Fig 1.16).

Bypass tracts may conduct either antegrade or retrograde. A premature atrial contraction that finds the accessory pathway refractory may pass through the AV node, capture the ventricle, conduct retrograde through the bypass tract, and establish a *reentrant circuit* with repetitive firing of the ventricles. Unlike other cases of reentry, there is no protected, reentrant focus (as in Fig 1.11).

When antegrade conduction and stimulation of the ventricles is through the AV node, the reentrant arrhythmia looks like PSVT with a narrow QRS complex (and, in fact, it is PSVT). A reentrant circuit in the opposite direction (see Fig 1.15), retrograde through the AV node and antegrade through the bypass tract, has a wide QRS complex because the sequence of ventricular activation is abnormal. It may look like ventricular tachycardia.

How can you tell whether this **wide QRS tachycardia** is ventricular or supraventricular? At times you cannot. The clinical setting helps. A young patient with a history of PSVT, no other heart disease, wide-complex tachycardia and no alteration of consciousness is likely to have PSVT with bypass tract reentry. An older patient with a history of heart failure or myocardial infarction, and who has had syncope or near syncope, should be treated assuming a diagnosis of ventricular tachycardia (VT). When in doubt, it is hard to go wrong treating the arrhythmia as probable VT. Direct current (DC) cardioversion is appropriate if the patient is unstable.

It is important to identify PSVT that is caused by pre-excitation, because the drug treatment is different. Digoxin, beta blockers, verapamil, and intravenous adenosine should be avoided because they slow AV nodal conduction, but not conduction through the bypass tract. If the patient develops atrial fibrillation or flutter, and drugs are used that slow AV node conduction, conduction through the bypass tract would be favored. Bypass tracts conduct more rapidly than the AV node: there could be a big increase in ventricular rate. Membrane-active agents, on the other hand, slow accessory pathway conduction; intravenous procainamide is the first choice for a patient with WPW who is having PSVT.

Procainamide has been used for long-term treatment of pre-excitation. The newest therapy is **catheter ablation** of bypass tracts, usually a cure. A catheter electrode is positioned next to the bypass tract, radiofrequency energy is applied, and the tissue touching the catheter is burned. Subsequent scarring effectively plugs the hole in the insulation. It is a relatively low-risk procedure and is better than life-long drug therapy, especially when drug therapy fails to prevent PSVT.

Sick Sinus Syndrome

The sick sinus syndrome is not just one arrhythmia, and it cannot be diagnosed on a single ECG. It is a group of different arrhythmias occurring at different times. It most commonly affects the elderly. There is usually SA node dysfunction, which causes profound bradycardia. The AV node may be sick as well, and the AV nodal escape rate during sinus bradycardia or SA arrest is inappropriately slow.

These patients with SA node dysfunction frequently have alternating bradycardia and supraventricular tachycardias. This seemingly paradoxical juxtaposition of slow and rapid heart rhythms has resulted in the term **brady-**

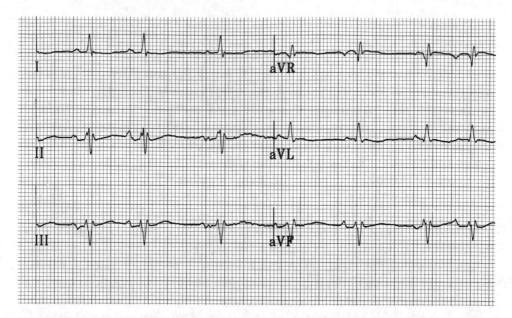

Figure 1.17 Wandering atrial pacemaker. These limb leads are from a patient with obstructive lung disease. The variation in P wave morphology is seen in lead II. Note the variable rate (RR interval). In the absence of obvious P waves before each QRS, this would look like atrial fibrillation. At rates above 100/min, wandering atrial pacemaker becomes multifocal atrial tachycardia (MAT).

tachy syndrome. The supraventricular tachycardias may include PSVT and atrial fibrillation and flutter. The patient may experience a variety of these arrhythmias, moving from one form of supraventricular tachycardia to another within a short time. Bouts of tachycardia may be followed by disturbingly long SA pauses with syncope. Diagnosis of the syndrome thus requires demonstrating a variety of these arrhythmias in a patient who has dizziness or syncope.

One interesting feature of the syndrome is that the medicines needed to control the rapid rhythms (e.g., digitalis, beta adrenergic blockers, calcium channel blockers) may aggravate the bradyarrhythmia. Treatment may thus combine pacing (to prevent bradycardia) and drug therapy (to prevent tachycardia).

Wandering Atrial Pacemaker and Multifocal Atrial Tachycardia

The rhythm of both wandering atrial pacemaker and multifocal atrial tachycardia (MAT) may be irregular; there are P waves before most QRS complexes, and the P waves have varying morphology (Fig 1.17). (Some feel that you should identify three different P wave morphologies before making the diagnosis.) The P waves apparently originate from varying sites in the atria. The difference between the terms is in the heart rate: when it is rapid, the second term (MAT) is used. Both are common arrhythmiae in patients with obstructive lung disease.

Ventricular Arrhythmias

Premature Ventricular Contractions

Most of us have premature ventricular contractions (PVC's), and they are a common finding on routine ECGs (Fig 1.18). Because they originate within the body of one of the ventricles, activation of the two ventricles is not simultaneous and the QRS is wide. PVC's and other ventricular rhythms may come from an **automatic focus,** tissue that is insulated from the surrounding muscle and that fires automatically at a fixed rate. When it discharges between heartbeats, when the surrounding muscle has repolarized and can be stimulated (is *vulnerable*), it produces a PVC. On the other hand, when the ectopic focus discharges while the ventricle is depolarized or before it is repolarized (during a QRS or a T wave), it finds the ventricle *refractory* to stimulation, and there is no PVC. Interestingly, this is the way old-fashioned, fixed-rate pacemakers work: they click along at a regular rate, capturing the ventricle only when it is vulnerable.

A second, and probably more common, mechanism for ventricular beats is **reentry,** a term discussed previously in relation to PSVT (see Fig 1.11). The reentrant focus is within the body of the ventricle, possibly an area of fibrosis or ischemia. Current enters the focus, but it is insulated from surrounding tissue. Conduction through the reentrant focus is slow. By the time the wave of depolarization exits the focus, the surrounding ventricle has been repolarized and can be stimulated, causing the PVC. A circuit may develop with repetitive stimulation of the ventricle. Most cases of ventricular tachycardia are thought to be reentrant rhythms. By convention, we often refer to extra beats or abnormal rhythms as **ectopic,** regardless of the mechanism (automatic or reentrant focus).

When reading ECGs, a common dilemma is deciding whether an ectopic beat is a PVC or is a PAC that is aberrantly conducted because of a blocked nerve below the AV node. **Aberrant conduction** produces a QRS complex that is wide and hard to distinguish from a PVC. One cause of wide-complex tachycardia is PSVT with aberrant infranodal conduction.

There are a few characteristics that help to make the distinction between PVC's and PAC's with aberrancy. Aberrant PAC's distort the QRS less, and

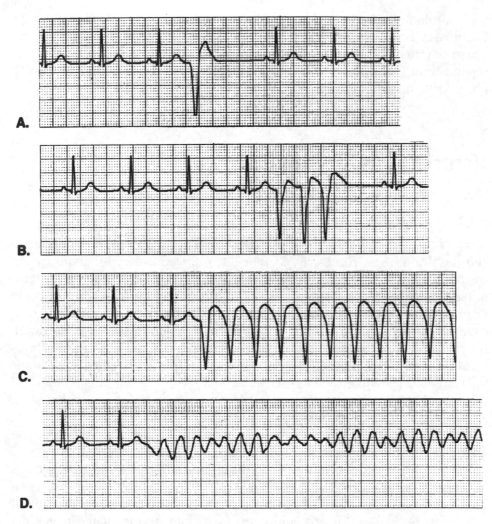

Figure 1.18 Ventricular arrhythmias. A: Isolated PVC. B: A ventricular triplet; ventricular tachycardia (VT) is defined as three or more PVC's in a row. C: Sustained VT. D: Ventricular fibrillation, the usual cause of sudden cardiac death.

Isolated PVC's are common in the absence of organic heart disease. More complex forms, including paired PVC's and VT, may be the consequence of LV dysfunction or acute ischemia.

the QRS axis tends to be similar to that of normal beats. That is to say, where normal beats have an upright (positive) QRS, the ectopic QRS is also upright. The PVC's T-wave axis is often opposite the QRS axis (i.e., when the QRS is positive, the T wave is negative). Aberrant conduction commonly affects the right bundle branch, which seems a weak link in the infranodal conduction system. Thus, aberrantly conducted PAC's often have a right bundle branch block pattern (see Chapter 2 for a description of right bundle branch block). Occasionally, the ectopic P wave can be seen distorting the preceding T wave, suggesting a PAC.

While helpful, these general characteristics are not totally reliable, and there is often uncertainty about the origin of extra beats.

Repetitive Ventricular Rhythms

Ventricular fibrillation is the usual cause of sudden cardiac death (see Fig 1.18). Frequent PVC's in a setting of *acute* MI indicate a high risk of ventricular fibrillation. With *chronic* heart disease, there is a hierarchy of ventricular arrhythmias, which may indicate a risk of sudden death (see Fig 1.18).

You must consider the risk of a ventricular arrhythmia in its clinical context. For example, patients with poor left ventricular function usually have *complex* ventricular arrhythmias and an increased risk of sudden cardiac death. Conversely, patients with complex arrhythmias often have poor left ventricular function.

A wide-complex tachycardia may be *ventricular tachycardia* (VT), but it may also be supraventricular tachycardia with aberrant conduction. Even rapid atrial fibrillation with associated bundle branch block can look like VT (although on close inspection, the rhythm is more irregular with AF). The clinical context is important in differentiating between VT and PSVT. Patients with acute MI or with a history of congestive heart failure are at high risk for developing VT. On the other hand, a young person without chest pain who is clinically stable—with the exception of palpitations—is more likely to have a supraventricular arrhythmia (perhaps even WPW, an example of an aberrantly conducted atrial rhythm). In this case, there may be a history of recurring, similar episodes.

The one ECG finding that allows you to diagnose VT with certainty is **AV dissociation.** During VT, if there is no retrograde conduction of ventricular impulses through the AV node to the atria (and there usually is not), the atria continue to beat independently. There are P waves clicking along at a regular rate that is slower than the VT rate, and these may be seen on the surface ECG (Fig 1.19). When electrophysiologists are unsure of the cause of wide-complex tachycardia, they record an ECG from within the right atrium. At this location, P waves are huge and easy to see: AV dissociation makes the diagnosis of VT.

Torsade de pointes is a curious form of ventricular tachycardia that is a favorite of Board examiners. The QRS complexes are polymorphic (variable) with an undulating pattern (Fig 1.20). The axis of each successive beat is different from the preceding one—the axis is "turning about a point." Conditions and drugs that cause QT interval prolongation may precipitate the arrhythmia. Most antiarrhythmic drugs have a paradoxical **proarrhythmic** ac-

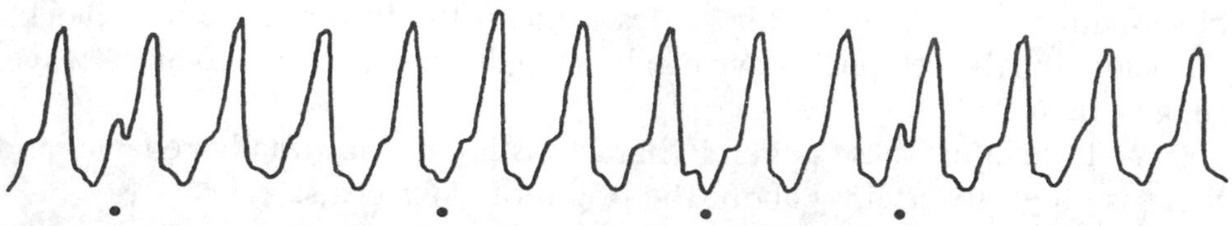

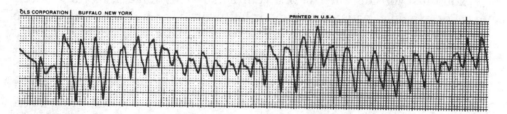

Figure 1.19 Ventricular tachycardia with AV dissociation. Finding intermittent P waves (marked with *dots*) that do not alter the ventricular rhythm is the most reliable indication that the tachycardia originates in the ventricle. If it originated in the atrium, there would necessarily be a relationship between atrial beats (P waves) and ventricular beats.

Figure 1.20 Torsade de pointes, an undulating, polymorphic VT in which the axis of each successive beat is different from that of the preceding one.

tion; torsade is the typical arrhythmia that may be caused by the class IA drugs (quinidine, procainamide, and disopyramide). It may be prevented by avoiding other conditions that prolong the QT interval (hypokalemia and hypomagnesemia), as well as by *combinations* of drugs that lengthen the QT (see Table 1.2).

Torsade is important to recognize, because its treatment is different from that of other forms of VT. Measures that shorten the QT interval are most effective. Intravenous magnesium often works. Increasing the heart rate also shortens the QT (with either temporary pacing or intravenous isoproterenol infusion).

Electrical Axis

The wave of depolarization passes through the heart in three dimensions, but each two-pole ECG lead records these events in just one dimension. Having 12 leads that are grouped in horizontal or frontal (vertical) planes allows us to reconstruct these events into three-dimensional space (see Fig 1.2). We are able to determine the spatial orientation, or *axis*, of each electrical event in the cardiac cycle.

Atrial depolarization starts high in the right atrium and moves down and to the left, toward the AV node (see Fig 1.3). The general direction, or axis, of the P wave is thus about 60° in the frontal plane. Because ECG lead II has its positive pole at 60° (see Fig 1.2), we would expect the P wave to be positive in that lead, and to have its maximum deflection or current in that lead. Lead aVR, with an orientation of −150°, would be expected to have a negative P wave.

What about the P wave in lead aVL, oriented just 90° from lead II? Simple vector principles tell us that measuring a vector from a perpendicular position produces a net measurement of zero. That is to say, the forces moving toward the position of measurement are balanced by the forces moving away. In lead aVL, the normal P wave either has little amplitude or is *biphasic*, with negative and positive deflections that are similar (in effect, canceling each other).

P wave axis is not usually measured; as long as it is positive in inferior leads, it is good enough. When it is negative in those leads, it indicates an ectopic atrial pacemaker located in the lower part of the atrium and depolarizing the atrium from bottom to top. This has little clinical significance, but it is worth comment when reading ECGs.

QRS Axis

From the AV node, the wave of depolarization moves first to the interventricular septum, discharging it from left to right, then through the body of the two ventricles (see Fig 1.3). The left ventricle is much thicker than the right and produces more voltage. The net vector of ventricular depolarization is therefore down and/or to the left in the frontal plane, normally about 60°, but ranging from 30° to +110°.

Measurement of the QRS axis in the frontal plane is a technical challenge for most students. It is not that hard, and the practice ECGs will help you to learn to do it quickly. The ECG computer measures the QRS axis with the simple principle of vector addition (Fig 1.21). You can easily do that with graph paper, and it is accurate, but there are faster ways.

One quick and simple method uses the principle that the QRS amplitude will be maximum and positive in the lead whose orientation is closest to the axis of the QRS vector. Thus, if the QRS axis is 0°, the QRS should have maximum amplitude in lead I. If the QRS axis is 90°, maximum amplitude should be in lead aVF. If leads I and aVF are both positive and with equal amplitude, the QRS should be half-way between them, or 45°. It is a crude approach, but at least it allows you to place the QRS vector within a quadrant.

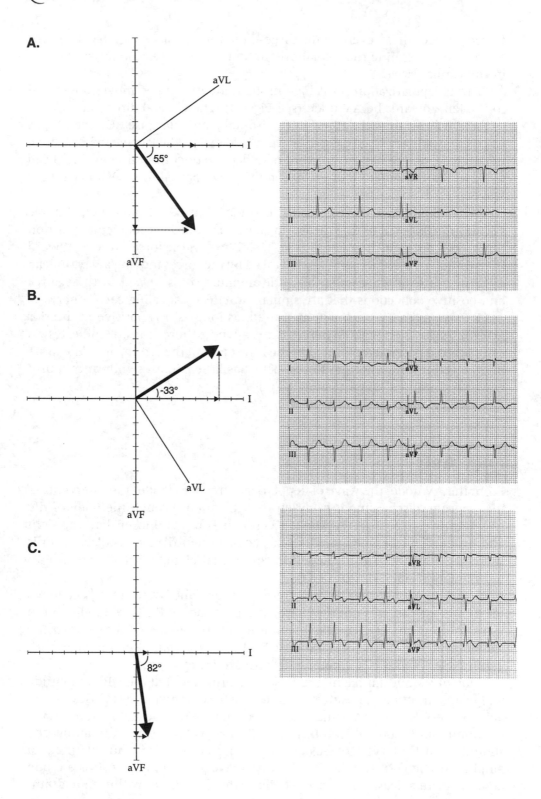

Another method uses the principle that a net vector amplitude of zero indicates that the direction of the vector is perpendicular (90°) to the voltmeter's orientation. Thus, if the positive and negative QRS deflections are equal, that is to say *isoelectric* (or add up to zero) in lead I of the ECG, the QRS vector is pointed at either +90° or −90°. If the QRS is positive in lead aVF, the axis must be +90°.

That is the method I use. I find a lead where the positive and negative QRS deflections are equal—where the QRS is isoelectric. *The QRS axis is perpendicular to that lead;* 90° in a direction that is quickly determined by looking at the general direction of the QRS vector (Fig 1.21).

It may not be possible to find an isoelectric lead for which positive and negative deflections are equal. In this case, I choose a lead for which the deflection is close to isoelectric. For example, if the positive forces in lead aVL are slightly, but not much higher than the negative forces, the axis is close

◀───

Figure 1.21 Calculation of the QRS axis: three examples. Vector addition is a simple process. Choose any two leads (the figure uses leads I and aVF) and plot the net voltage. Move one of these plotted vectors so that its tail is positioned at the head of the other (*dotted line*). The sum of vector addition is the line drawn from the origin to the head of the repositioned vector (*bold line*). This is the mean QRS vector, and the axis can be measured with a protractor.

There are faster ways to estimate the QRS vector. Look first at example C. In lead I, the positive and negative forces almost cancel each other; net voltage is just 0.1 mV (1 mm). When this tiny vector is moved to aVF, the resulting mean QRS vector is quite close to aVF. If the net forces in lead I equaled 0 mV (i.e., lead I was isoelectric), there would have been no displacement of the mean vector from aVF at all. The final QRS axis would be 90°. This illustrates the method I use for estimating the QRS axis: find a lead where the QRS is isoelectric (or close to isoelectric). The QRS vector is perpendicular to that lead.

Try this for the other two examples. A: The QRS is isoelectric in lead aVL; 90° from aVL is +60°, and that is the QRS vector. Why is it not −120°, 90° in the other direction from aVL? Simply because the QRS is positive in the right lower quadrant leads (I, II, aVF). B: The QRS is almost isoelectric in II; 90° from II is either −30° or +150°. Because the QRS is positive in the left side-leads (I and aVL), the axis is close to −30°. Actually, the net forces in II are slightly negative, which pushes the vector a little farther to the left. I am calling the axis −35°, identifying this as left axis deviation (LAD).

to 60°, but actually a little more in the direction of aVL (perhaps 55°). It is a good approximation.

As you work through the first of the practice ECGs, we will pay close attention to measuring the QRS axis.

T Wave Axis

The T wave axis, like the P wave axis, is not usually calculated. Generally, it is in the same direction as the QRS axis. Where the QRS is positive, the T wave is also positive. T wave inversion—a T wave axis opposite that of the QRS—is an abnormal finding that will be discussed in the next chapter.

2

Morphologic Changes in P, QRS, ST, and T

You have recorded rate, rhythm, intervals, and the QRS axis. The next step in reading the ECG is to evaluate the P wave, QRS complex, ST segment, and T wave for abnormalities, and then give a final interpretation. This is an exercise in pattern recognition. Yet ECG changes logically reflect what is happening with the heart's anatomy and physiology. All of it makes more sense if you think of mechanism while learning diagnostic criteria.

Atrial (P Wave) Abnormalities

Left Atrial Abnormality

There are two possible patterns of left atrial abnormality (LAA). The most common is a *biphasic P wave in lead* V_1 (Fig 2.1). For it to be significant, the negative deflection has to be deep enough and wide enough to contain a small box (i.e., 1×1 mm).

LAA is seen with conditions that increase left ventricular diastolic pressure—and therefore left atrial pressure—including congestive heart failure and left ventricular hypertrophy. One study found that LAA was the earliest ECG indicator of hypertensive heart disease, appearing well before other features of left ventricular hypertrophy. It may be a transient finding; I have seen it during acute pulmonary edema, and then found it gone on the next day's tracing after diuresis (and reduction of left atrial pressure).

39

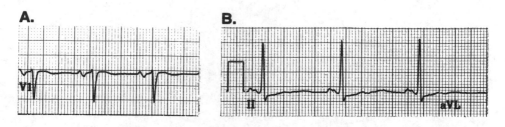

Figure 2.1 Left atrial abnormality (LAA). Two ECG findings may be used to make the diagnosis. A: Biphasic P wave in lead V₁; the negative deflection should be 1 mm deep and wide. B: Broad, notched P wave in one of the limb leads, most commonly II, III, or aVF, as the P wave vector is aimed at the inferior leads.

The second LAA pattern is a *broad, notched P wave* in one of the limb leads (usually in lead II, III, or aVF) (see Fig 2.1). This develops in patients with marked dilatation of the left atrium, as may be seen with mitral stenosis or regurgitation ("P mitrale").

Right Atrial Abnormality

Normally, P waves are less than 2.5 mm tall (in any lead). In right atrial abnormality (RAA), the P waves are tall and narrow, and they appear peaked (Fig 2.2). *P amplitude ≥2.5 mm* in those leads oriented along the P wave axis

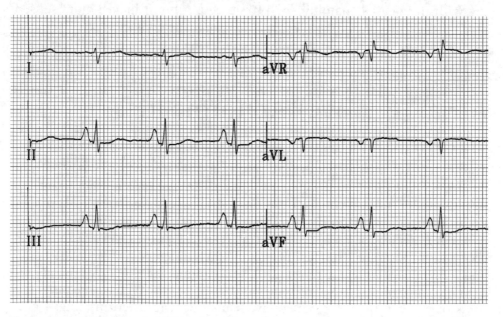

Figure 2.2 Right atrial abnormality (RAA). Tall, peaked P waves in inferior leads (at least 2.5 mm in one of the leads).

(the inferior limb leads, II, III, and aVF) usually indicates RAA. This often is referred to as P pulmonale, because it may be caused by advanced lung disease with associated pulmonary artery hypertension. It is seen with pulmonary hypertension caused by congenital heart disease as well.

Intraventricular Conduction Abnormalities

Normally, the wave of depolarization exits the bundle of His, moves through the two bundle branches, and activates the two ventricles *simultaneously* (see Fig 1.3). When one of the bundle branches, or one of their major divisions, is injured and conduction is blocked, the affected ventricular region is stimulated late by current that has spread from an adjacent ventricular region. Late activation creates a deflection at the terminal end of the QRS complex, making the overall QRS complex wider. A QRS duration of 0.12 sec or more (3 mm) is the basic diagnostic criterion for bundle branch block.

Right Bundle Branch Block

When the right bundle branch is blocked (RBBB), the interventricular septum and the left ventricle are activated normally (Fig 2.3). Current then spreads from the left to the right ventricle, which is depolarized late. Electrical events that occur early—septal and left ventricular activation—are thus unchanged. What is different is an extra deflection at the end of the QRS caused by late, right ventricular depolarization.

I will restate this with reference to specific changes on the ECG. But first, recall a basic principle of electrocardiography regarding the polarity of leads. Each lead has spatial orientation and polarity (see Fig 1.2). A wave of depolarization that moves toward the positive pole of a lead produces a positive (upright) deflection, an R wave. That is to say, if the vector of the wave of depolarization is in the direction of the lead, the deflection is positive. If the wave of depolarization moves away from the positive and toward the negative pole of a lead, it still is detected, but it produces a negative (downward) deflection, an S wave.

Back to RBBB (see Fig 2.3): Lead V_1, on the *right side* of the chest, sits just over the right ventricle (RV) and is a sensitive detector of right ventricular events. In RBBB, lead V_1 first records normal septal activation (a positive deflection, or R wave, because the septum depolarizes from left to right), then normal left ventricular activation (a negative deflection, or S wave, as the

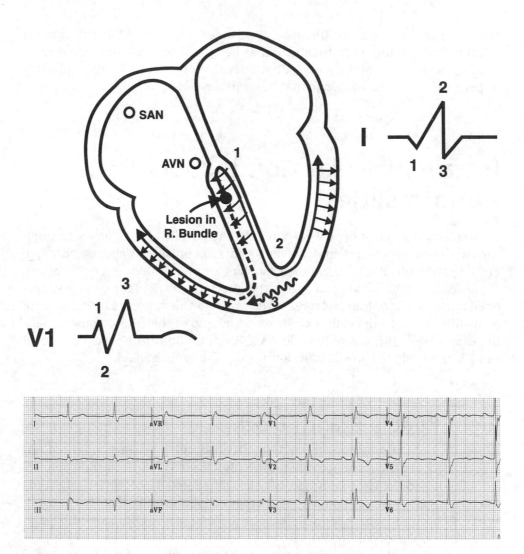

Figure 2.3 Right bundle branch block (RBBB). A: Follow the sequence of ventricular activation, and its effect on leads I and V₁, which, in the figure, are appropriately positioned. 1) There is normal septal activation from left to right. 2) Left ventricular activation is normal. 3) Because the right bundle branch is blocked, current must move from the left ventricle to the right, and this occurs late. The tail-end of the QRS is slurred because of late depolarization of the right side. **B:** Pattern recognition: RSR in V₁ + wide QRS.

wave of depolarization moves posteriorly and to the left through the left ven-tricle [LV]). Finally, current works its way from the LV to the RV—remember, it could not get there directly because of the blocked right bundle. *The vector of RV depolarization is aimed at V_1*; thus, the terminal deflection in V_1 is positive (upright), another R wave. RBBB thus produces an RSR' pattern in V_1. In other leads, terminal forces (the RV vector) also are oriented toward the right. Thus, terminal QRS forces in left-side leads, such as I, aVL, and V_6, would be negative (an S wave).

RBBB Recognition   RSR pattern in V_1, and QRS ≥ 0.12 sec.

Incomplete Right Bundle Branch Block

Diagnosis   RSR' pattern in V_1, and QRS duration <0.12 sec.

Incomplete right bundle branch block (IRBBB) is usually a normal vari-ant, but in some cases it reflects RV hypertrophy or dilatation. Our ECG com-puter program interprets it as "RV volume overload." IRBBB is a common, almost invariable, finding with atrial septal defect (ASD), in which the RV may pump 2 or 3 times as much blood as the LV. ASD may cause no symp-toms until a person reaches age 50. The diagnosis of IRBBB may be suggested on a routine ECG. A young person with IRBBB should at least have a good physical exam and chest x-ray, and an echocardiogram if these screening studies are abnormal. (ASD causing IRBBB, by the way, has been a favorite of Board examiners in internal medicine and cardiology.)

Left Bundle Branch Block

In left bundle branch block (LBBB), the sequence of ventricular activation is almost the opposite of that described with RBBB. The left bundle innervates the interventricular septum, so initial septal depolarization, normally from left to right, is lost (Fig 2.4). The initial small negative deflection in left-side leads (I, aVL, V_6) is lost—the so-called septal Q wave. The septum is instead activated from right to left, causing an initial positive deflection in left-side leads. Because the right ventricle is thin walled, little current is produced by RV excitation. Septal and early left ventricular activation predominate, and current generated by RV discharge (which would be oriented anterior and to the right) is buried within the LV complex. LV activation is slow because of the blocked left bundle, and the QRS complex is wide. The terminal forces are aimed at the blocked side, to the left; therefore, the terminal portion of the QRS is positive in left-side leads such as I, aVL, and V_6 (see Fig 2.4).

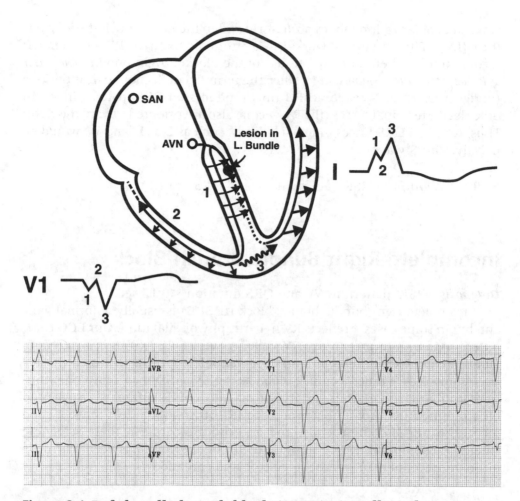

Figure 2.4 Left bundle branch block (LBBB). A: Follow the
sequence of ventricular activation. 1) The normal left-to-right
depolarization of the septum is interrupted by the blocked left
bundle branch. The septum is activated from right to left. 2)
Activation of the thin-walled RV produces little current. 3) The LV
is depolarized late by current working its way over from the right
side, and terminal QRS forces are oriented toward the left. **B:**
Pattern recognition: broad positive complex—often notched—in
left-side leads (I, aVL). Small Q waves in these leads would
exclude LBBB because they would indicate normal, left-to-right
activation of the septum. This patient also had marked LAD. T
wave changes and prolongation of the QT interval may accompany
LBBB. It is not possible to diagnose either LVH or MI in the
presence of LBBB (see later).

Diagnosis of LBBB   Broad, positive complex in left-side leads (I, aVL, and V₆), with the QRS duration ≥0.12 sec (3 mm).

Left Anterior and Posterior Fascicular Block

The fascicular blocks, or **hemiblocks,** cause changes in the QRS axis. The left bundle divides into anterior and posterior branches, or fascicles. The *anterior fascicle* is a thin nerve that runs through the septum close to the right bundle branch. It is relatively susceptible to injury, possibly because of its size and location, and left anterior fascicular block (LAFB) is common. The left *posterior fascicle* is a broad group of nerves that fans out through the posterior region of the interventricular septum. Possibly because of the space it occupies, it is less susceptible to injury than the anterior branch, and left posterior fascicular block (LPFB) is less common than LAFB.

Diagnostic criteria   The QRS complex is not necessarily wider than normal; the diagnosis is made when there is a *shift in axis.*

1.   LAFB: Extreme left-axis deviation, at least −45° not caused by inferior MI.

2.   LPFB: Right-axis deviation (RAD) >90° (some have suggested more extreme RAD, as much as 110° or 120°).

This is a bit oversimplified, as other conditions may cause a shift in QRS axis. The most common of these is inferior MI with deep Q waves in inferior leads and extreme left-axis deviation. Inferior infarction does not alter conduction through the left anterior fascicle. When there are inferior Q waves (reviewed later in this chapter), I diagnose left axis deviation rather than LAFB.

Bifascicular Block

Think of the infranodal system as having three branches, or fascicles: the right bundle and the two branches of the left bundle. LBBB, or block of both branches of the left bundle, could be considered bifascicular block. However, the term is usually reserved for RBBB plus block of one of the two branches of the left bundle (RBBB plus LAFB, or RBBB plus LPFB).

Because of the anatomic proximity of the right bundle and left anterior fascicle, conditions that injure one often affect the other; the combination of *RBBB plus LAFB* is observed in as many as 1 in 25 hospitalized patients. The diagnosis is simple: there is RBBB plus extreme left axis deviation (LAD). This condition does not necessarily reflect advanced, serious heart disease. A small amount of fibrosis may block the two nerves. Many patients with RBBB plus LAFB have normal LV function and no other structural cardiac abnormalities.

By contrast, patients with other forms of bifascicular block—RBBB plus LPFB, or LBBB—usually have detectable, structural problems, such as poor LV function, ischemic injury, or hypertrophy.

Ventricular Hypertrophy, QRS Amplitude, and R Wave Progression

First, the big picture; then we will get to the specifics. Pressure overload of a ventricle may be caused by increased vascular resistance downstream, or ventricular outflow tract obstruction. The ventricle responds to pressure overload by adding muscle, just as you add muscle to your arms with weight lifting. Increased muscle thickness on one side of the heart or the other may cause a shift in QRS axis toward the hypertrophied side and an increase in voltage (more muscle, more voltage).

The large coronary artery branches are located on the epicardial surface of the heart, and they send blood to underlying muscle through small perforating branches. An increase in ventricular thickness means an increase in the *distance* from the epicardial artery to the endocardium. Blood supply to the subendocardial region—farthest from the epicardial source—may be compromised, causing changes in the ST segment and T wave that look ischemic (and may be referred to as a *strain* pattern). It is as if the ventricle outgrows its blood supply. Most coronary blood flow occurs during diastole. The relative reduction in flow to subendocardial regions with hypertrophy is aggravated by high ventricular diastolic pressures.

Finally, high ventricular diastolic pressures are reflected back to the atria, causing atrial (P wave) abnormalities on the ECG.

Left Ventricular Hypertrophy

Predictably, left ventricular hypertrophy (LVH) causes an increase in LV voltage and ST segment and T wave changes in those leads with high voltage (the LV strain pattern), a shift in axis to the left, and LAA (Fig 2.5). In addition, there may be slight widening of the QRS to more than 0.09 sec, and some patients develop LBBB. However, LBBB changes the QRS complex enough that LVH cannot be diagnosed when LBBB is present. The initial upstroke of the R wave in V_5 and V_6, the **intrinsicoid deflection,** may be prolonged to over 0.04 sec. This is the time that it takes the LV to be activated, and it is longer when the ventricle is thickened.

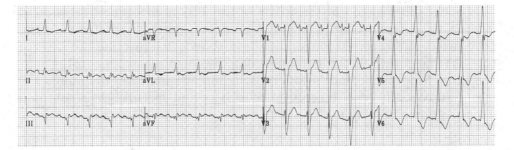

Figure 2.5 Left ventricular hypertrophy (LVH). This patient with aortic stenosis had LAA, high QRS voltage (V_2), ST-T changes in lateral leads (the typical LV strain pattern), and wide QRS. He did not have LAD, and the intrinsicoid deflection was on the borderline (see Table 2.1).

A patient with LVH may not have all these ECG findings, especially early in the development of LVH (see Fig 2.5). The diagnosis can be made when just some of these features are present, but with fewer findings, the accuracy of the diagnosis is lower. The Estes scoring system is provided in Table 2.1. A point total of 5 makes the diagnosis of LVH, and with 4 points, the patient has probable LVH. Using multiple diagnostic criteria rather than QRS voltage alone gives good specificity (fewer false positives, less overdiagnosis).

Table 2.1 The Estes Point System for Left Ventricular Hypertrophy (LVH)

1. Amplitude .... 3 points
   Any of the following
      (a) Largest R or S wave in the limb leads $\geq$ 20 mm
      (b) S wave in V_1 or V_2 $\geq$ 30 mm
      (c) R wave in V_5 or V_6 $\geq$ 30 mm

2. ST-T changes (typical pattern of left ventricular strain with the ST segment vector shifted in direction opposite to the mean QRS vector)
   Without digitalis .... 3 points
   With digitalis .... 1 point

3. Left atrial abnormality .... 3 points

4. Left axis deviation ($-30°$ or more) .... 2 points

5. QRS duration $\geq$ 0.09 sec .... 1 point

6. Intrinsicoid deflection in V_5 and V_6 $\geq$ 0.05 sec .... 1 point

---

LVH = 5 or more points
Probable LVH = 4 points

On the other hand, the sensitivity of the ECG in detecting LVH is poor; it tends to underdiagnose. Using an ECG point system, both anatomic and echocardiographic correlation studies have shown that just half the cases of true LVH meet rigid ECG criteria. Relaxing the diagnostic criteria, using voltage alone for example, increases sensitivity but also increases the number of false positives. This choice between sensitivity and specificity is a common dilemma when reading ECGs.

Sermonette   Avoid overdiagnosis. LVH demonstrates the importance of this principle. Young people often have high QRS voltage, particularly if thin or athletic. Using voltage, alone, to diagnose LVH could mean assigning that diagnosis to healthy young people. LVH is considered bad heart disease, and that diagnosis would create a serious problem for anyone applying for a job or for insurance. It seems better to stick with strict ECG diagnostic criteria for LVH, recognizing the insensitivity of the ECG.

Counter-sermon   LVH is a serious heart condition. For example, patients with coronary artery disease who also have LVH have a worse prognosis. Any ECG finding that would lead to earlier diagnosis and treatment would justify the risks of overdiagnosis.

In most cases, I place my vote for specificity (first, do no harm).

Right Ventricular Hypertrophy

Normally, most of the voltage in the QRS complex is generated by the LV, which is much thicker than the RV. This makes the QRS complex in the right-side precordial leads (V_1 and V_2) negative, and positive in the left-side precordial leads (V_4 through V_6). The *transition* from negative to positive complexes usually occurs around V_3–V_4. That changes with right ventricular hypertrophy (RVH). As you would expect, RVH causes an increase in RV voltage over the right chest leads, and an associated shift in QRS axis toward the right. There is often a strain pattern in leads reflecting high RV voltage (Fig 2.6). Specific diagnostic criteria are outlined in Table 2.2.

RVH may not cause all these changes. The voltage changes alone may be used to make the diagnosis. I feel more confident when there is also ST-T change or axis shift. The possibility of false positives is enough that I usually hedge when reading ECGs with no clinical history ("possible RVH"). On the other hand, in the presence of a condition that may cause RVH (e.g., obstructive lung disease with probable cor pulmonale, mitral valve or congenital heart disease with pulmonary hypertension, or pulmonary stenosis), finding the typical ECG pattern points to RVH. Unfortunately, the absence of the ECG findings does not exclude RVH.

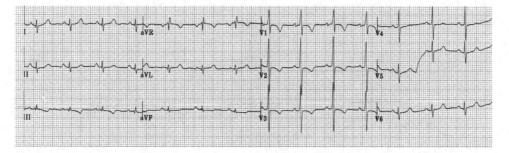

Figure 2.6 Right ventricular hypertrophy (RVH). This young woman with primary pulmonary hypertension had rightward axis, tall R in V$_1$, deep S in V$_6$, and ST-T changes in the right precordial leads (the RV strain pattern). She did not have RAA (see Table 2.2).

Delayed, or Poor, R Wave Progression in Precordial Leads

To this point, each section has considered a cardiac diagnosis. This and a number of following sections will consider ECG findings that do not clearly indicate anatomic or functional abnormalities, and that must be recognized in the interpretation as nonspecific.

As noted previously, negative (S wave) forces predominate over right chest (precordial) leads. There is *transition* in the midprecordial leads, and the QRS should be isoelectric (with positive and negative forces equal) by lead V$_3$. In leads V$_4$ through V$_6$ the R wave amplitude should exceed negative forces. Delay in transition, or poor R wave progression, simply means that

---

Table 2.2 Diagnosis of Right Ventricular Hypertrophy

Criteria
    R/S in V$_1$ ≥ 1, or
    R in V$_1$ ≥ 7 mm, or
    R in V$_1$ + S in V$_5$ or V$_6$ > 10.5 mm

Supportive findings
    Right axis deviation ≥ 110°
    Right atrial abnormality (RAA)
    ST depression + T wave inversion in V$_1$ or V$_2$ (RV strain)

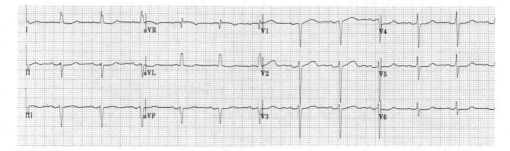

Figure 2.7 Poor R wave progression (PRWP). Transition from a negative to positive QRS complex normally happens by lead V$_4$. This patient's QRS is still negative in V$_4$ and V$_5$.

this transition point is further to the left (Fig 2.7), and that most of the precordial leads have (net) negative voltage.

Delay in transition is not a diagnosis, just a description of the ECG changes. *Chronic obstructive pulmonary disease (COPD)* is such a common cause that our computer is programmed to call poor R wave progression (PRWP) a pulmonary pattern when there is associated low QRS voltage. I always change that to PRWP of unknown cause. Think for a moment of COPD with its barrel-chest deformity. On chest x-ray, the heart may appear to be hanging more vertically in the hyperexpanded chest cavity, and on physical exam the apical impulse is best felt in the subxiphoid region. As part of this shift in position within the chest, there appears to be rotation of the heart clockwise, to the left, so that the LV is more posterior and to the left than usual. This change in position usually is responsible for PRWP in patients with COPD.

On the other hand, COPD can cause cor pulmonale with RVH. This may cause deep S waves in V$_5$ and V$_6$ just like PRWP due to the change in cardiac position. Remember that RVH also causes tall R waves in V$_1$, which I think of as the RV lead. Studies correlating ECG and anatomic findings have shown that a diagnosis of RVH with a deep S wave in V$_6$ but no tall R waves in V$_1$ is associated with more false positives.

Other conditions

1. LV dilatation, as seen with pure volume overload such as mitral regurgitation, may displace the LV (and apical impulse) far to the left. In this case, the precordial leads may not overlie the body of the LV until positions V$_5$ or V$_6$, causing a delay in R wave progression.

2. LAFB is commonly associated with PRWP in the absence of other cardiac conditions.

3. Anterior MI causes a loss of positive forces in anterior precordial leads, and PRWP.

4. A final and common cause of delayed R progression is misplacement of the chest leads.

Low QRS Voltage

Diagnostic criterion   The QRS amplitude is less than 5 mm in all of the limb leads. When this is the case, the amplitude in each of the precordial (V) leads is usually less than 10 mm, but that is not necessary for the diagnosis.

As with PRWP, low voltage should be considered a description, not a diagnosis. It may be a normal variant. Among the cardiac conditions associated with low QRS voltage are dilated cardiomyopathy, infiltrative cardiomyopathy (e.g., amyloidosis), pericardial effusion, and constrictive pericarditis. Noncardiac causes include hypothyroidism, emphysema, and obesity. Low voltage is such a nonspecific finding that it is not considered a diagnostic criterion for any of these illnesses.

ST Segment and T Wave Changes and Q Waves: Patterns of Ischemia and Infarction

Myocardial ischemia tends to be a regional event (Fig 2.8). Only one of the major coronaries is likely to cause ischemia or infarction at a time. To have multiple branches develop stenoses that cause active ischemia *simultaneously* would be a rare coincidence. Thus, an ischemic event is limited to the *anterior* wall (the anterior descending artery, the precordial V leads), the *inferior* wall (usually the right coronary artery, ECG leads II, III, and aVF), or the *lateral* wall (the circumflex artery, leads I, aVL, and V_6).

There can be some overlap in vascular distributions, as there is considerable anatomic variation among people. Thus, occlusion of an especially large right coronary artery that loops around to the lateral wall might cause *inferolateral* infarction with ECG changes in inferior leads, plus changes in one or more of the lateral leads. A large anterior descending artery might have branches that supply part of the lateral wall, and *anterolateral* MI would mean changes in anterior precordial leads plus one or more of the lateral leads (see Fig 2.8).

ECG changes that are global, involving all the vascular regions, are rarely caused by ischemia. Pericarditis, for example, affects the entire heart and causes ST segment and T wave changes that are **global** (present in anterior, inferior, and lateral leads).

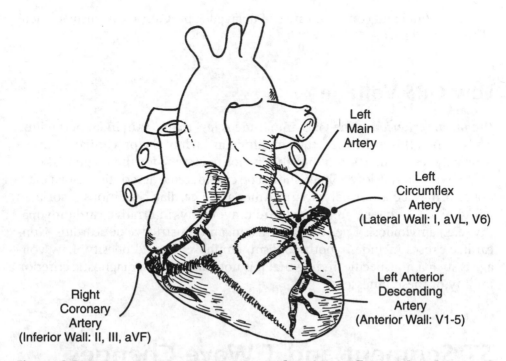

Figure 2.8 Coronary artery anatomy. The circumflex and right coronary arteries circle the heart in the AV groove; branches of the circumflex leave the groove to supply the lateral wall, and the major right coronary branch (the posterior descending artery), supplies the inferior wall. The anterior descending artery is located just over the interventricular septum (the *interventricular groove*); it sends perforating branches into the septum, and diagonal branches to the anterior LV surface. The spatial orientation of the ECG leads allows groups of leads to be particularly sensitive to events in a given region of the heart (see Fig 1.2 as well).

MI and injury cause a variety of changes in ST segments, T waves, and the QRS complex. The following section is organized around the ECG changes. While reading this, you may find it useful to refer to Table 2.3, which organizes the same ECG findings according to cardiac diagnoses—same information, just a different way of looking at it.

ST Segment Depression

During the short time from the end of the QRS complex to the beginning of the T wave, no voltage is recorded by the ECG; the ST segment is isoelectric (see Fig 1.2). (Note that **isoelectric** can mean that there is no voltage—as

Table 2.3 ECG Changes with Syndromes of Myocardial Ischemia

CONDITION	ECG CHANGES	TIMING	PATHOPHYSIOLOGY
Angina pectoris	ST Depression	Coincidental with chest pain	Stenosed artery, but with some antegrade flow; O$_2$ demand exceeds supply; subendocardial ischemia
Coronary artery spasm (angina pectoris)	ST Elevation	Coincidental with chest pain	Spasm may occur in a normal artery or at the site of plaque; usually total occlusion; transmural ischemia, temporary
Non-Q MI	ST Depression	During pain	Stenosed artery, but with some antegrade flow; subendocardial ischemia, then necrosis
	T Wave Inversion	May be permanent	
Q Wave MI	ST Elevation	Coincidental with pain	Total occlusion, transmural ischemia, then necrosis
	T Wave Inversion	Minutes to hours later, while ST elevation persists	
	Q Wave	Minutes to hours after onset of MI; permanent	

is the case with the ST segment that rests on the baseline—or it can mean that positive and negative forces are equal, canceling each other with a net sum of zero.)

A shift in the ST segment from the baseline may indicate ischemia. **ST depression** occurs with **subendocardial ischemia** (Fig 2.9). Cardiac catheterization during subendocardial ischemia usually reveals that the coronary artery supplying the ischemic zone is tightly stenosed, but not (totally) occluded. There is a mismatch between blood supply and demand across the stenosed artery, and the region of myocardium farthest from the epicardial artery—the subendocardium—is the most ischemic.

The ECG in Fig 2.10 is a good example. It was recorded during a treadmill stress test from a middle-aged woman with chronic, stable angina pectoris. At rest, she had no ST segment depression. During exercise, heart rate and

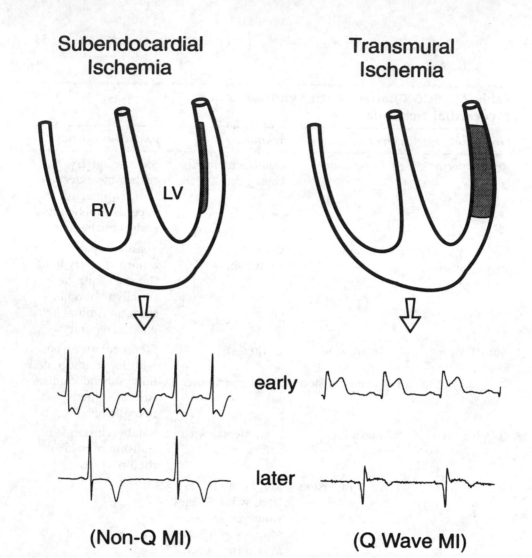

Subendocardial Ischemia

Transmural Ischemia

RV   LV

early

later

(Non-Q MI)

(Q Wave MI)

Figure 2.9 Patterns of myocardial ischemia. The epicardium is the outside surface of the heart, and the endocardium is the surface next to the ventricular cavity. The coronary arteries are located on the epicardial surface. Subendocardial *(nontransmural)* ischemia causes ST segment depression. If ischemia persists, and there is myocardial injury, there may be T wave inversion (a pattern called subendocardial or nontransmural or non-Q wave infarction). Transmural ischemia is caused by total occlusion of the artery. During acute ischemia, there is ST segment elevation. Resolution of spasm or dissolution of thrombus may open the occluded artery before there is injury. In this case, the episode of ischemia represents angina pectoris. If occlusion and, therefore, ischemia persist and there is myocardial injury, the pattern is called *transmural* or *Q wave infarction.*

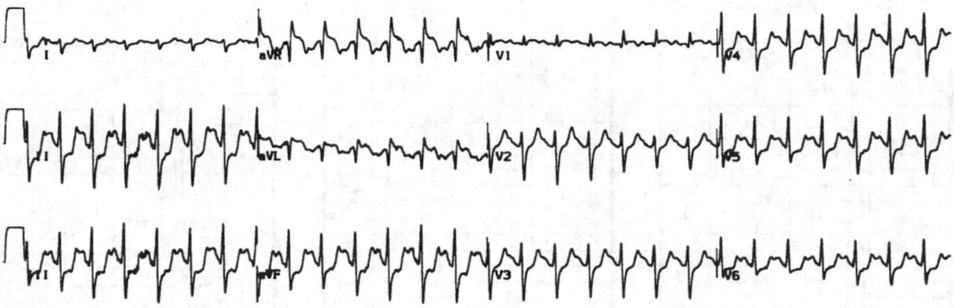

Figure 2.10 Positive stress ECG. At rest, the patient's ECG was normal. While walking on the treadmill, she developed ST segment depression (inferior and lateral leads). Within 3 minutes, she experienced chest heaviness, and exercise was stopped.

systemic blood pressure rose, both in direct proportion to the increase in cardiac work. Increased cardiac work means an increase in myocardial oxygen demand. To meet the increase in oxygen demand, her coronary artery blood flow increased. But the coronary artery stenosis placed a limit on how much the arterial blood flow could increase. When cardiac work load exceeded that limit, she developed ST segment depression and angina pectoris.

That is the pathophysiology of **chronic, stable angina:** a mismatch between oxygen supply and demand across a fixed coronary artery stenosis. An increase in oxygen demand (e.g., exercise or stress) usually precipitates angina, and reduced demand (e.g., rest, nitrates, or beta adrenergic blockers) provides relief.

During ischemia, the ST segments are depressed well below baseline (see Fig 2.10). In addition, the ST segments have a check-mark or hockey-stick appearance, and the segments are either horizontal or downsloping (Fig 2.11). This is the typical shape of ST segments depressed by acute ischemia. A depressed but up-sloping ST segment is not as specific for ischemia (see Fig 2.11). In this case, the **J point**—the junction between the QRS complex and the beginning of the ST segment—is depressed below the baseline, but the ST segment moves rapidly upward.

Poor specificity is a fundamental problem with the diagnosis of subendocardial ischemia based on ST depression. Other conditions may cause ST depression including LVH, digitalis, and hypokalemia. It is a common finding in older patients both with and without a history of ischemic heart disease. ST depression on a routine ECG does not necessarily indicate the presence of coronary artery stenosis, and in the absence of any clinical history you should consider it a nonspecific finding. Associated T wave flattening and inversion are common; their presence does not change the fact that the findings are nonspecific.

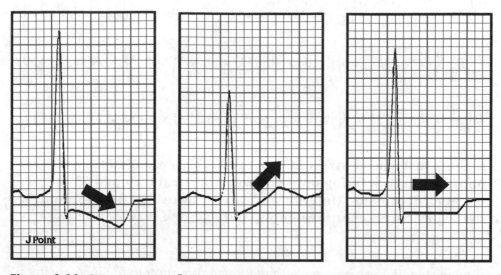

Figure 2.11 ST segment depression. The J point is the junction of the QRS complex and the beginning of the ST segment. Downsloping and horizontal ST depression are more specific for subendocardial ischemia than is J point depression with upsloping ST's.

Nonspecific ST-T wave changes (**NSST-TCs,** according to our Heart Station secretary) is a frequently applied ECG interpretation. Do not be frustrated by this or consider it a cop-out; instead, accept it as the interpretation of a sophisticated reader who understands the limitations of the ECG.

When is ST depression specific (that is to say, diagnostic)? When it is placed in the clinical context. The stress test is a good example (see Fig 2.10). An ECG obtained during chest pain and that can be *compared with a previous tracing* is another. For a patient with chest pain of uncertain etiology, finding ST depression *during pain* may make the diagnosis of angina pectoris. The absence of ST segment changes with pain makes coronary disease less likely.

T Wave Inversion

T wave inversion may be observed *during* acute ischemia (that is to say, during chest pain), and it is often associated with ST segment changes, either depression or elevation. T inversion that develops during chest pain, like ST depression, is evidence of a cardiac etiology. It may also be a permanent finding after pain has resolved. In that case, T inversion indicates *myocardial infarction* (permanent injury with loss of muscle and scar formation). Deep, symmetrical T inversion is the ECG finding of **non-Q wave infarction,** also called **nontransmural** or **subendocardial infarction** (Fig 2.12).

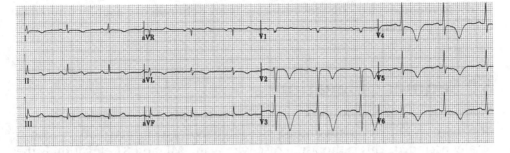

Figure 2.12 Anterior, non-Q MI. This may be called *subendocardial* **or** *nontransmural MI.* **There is deep and symmetrical T wave inversion in the anterior leads. Note that the QT interval is long; this is not a criterion for non-Q MI, but may accompany it (and indicates increased risk of ventricular arrhythmias).**

Let us backtrack a moment and be sure that we understand the sequence of events with ischemia (see Table 2.3 and Fig 2.9). It is the direction of ST segment shift that distinguishes subendocardial from transmural ischemia. The combination of chest pain and ST depression indicates ongoing, subendocardial ischemia. If pain is prolonged, and there is myocardial injury, T wave inversion develops and may be permanent. Deep and symmetrical T wave inversion is the non-Q wave infarct pattern, and ST depression may resolve when the pain (active ischemia) is over. With non-Q wave infarction, injury is limited to the subendocardium, not the full thickness of the ventricle (see Fig 2.9). Cardiac catheterization during the acute phase of non-Q wave MI (during pain) shows that the infarct artery is tightly stenosed, but that there is still some antegrade flow.

With non-Q wave MI, the amount of injury is small compared with full-thickness, transmural, Q wave infarction (see Fig 2.9). That is good, as heart muscle is irreplaceable. But note that after non-Q MI, the patient still has the tightly stenosed artery and is at risk for future ischemic injury. Non-Q MI is usually considered an indication for cardiac catheterization and possible revascularization.

Nonischemic cardiac conditions, including pericarditis and virtually any disease that affects myocardium, may cause T wave inversion. Intracranial bleeding may cause deep T wave inversion; look for this on Board exams. The ECG recording in Figure 2.12 could be the result of intracranial hemorrhage. Pathologic studies have shown that most of these patients suffer subendocardial injury at the time of stroke—the T wave changes come from the heart, not the brain. Children and young adults may have T inversion, the so-called juvenile pattern.

Nonischemic heart disease, such as pericarditis, generally produce global changes, altering ST segments and T waves in anterior, inferior, and lateral leads. Remember that changes resulting from ischemia are usually limited to one vascular region.

ST Segment Elevation

The most common cause of ST elevation is transmural MI. Catheterization of patients with chest pain and ST elevation shows a coronary artery that is totally occluded. This is the usual case with acute MI, and ST elevation is the primary ECG indication for thrombolytic therapy or emergency angioplasty. Compared with ST segment depression, ST elevation is a more specific indicator of acute ischemia. Most patients with new ST elevation are in the emergency room with chest pain.

Vasospastic, or **Prinzmetal's, angina pectoris** also causes ST elevation. It is unusual to get an angiogram during a spontaneous episode, but it is possible to induce coronary spasm during cardiac catheterization using ergonovine. During pain with ST elevation, these patients usually have total coronary occlusion. Note the basic differences between this and chronic stable angina. Spasm is a dynamic lesion, and the event initiating ischemia is a reduction in blood flow. Chronic stable angina involves a fixed stenosis; the event initiating ischemia is not a spontaneous reduction in blood flow but instead an increase in myocardial oxygen demand (exercise).

Acute MI with ST segment elevation is a dramatic finding on the ECG (Figs 2.13, 2.14). ST elevation may be called the **current of injury.** Review these tracings from seven patients with inferior or anterior MI. ST elevation is lim-

---

▶

Figure 2.13 Four patients with acute inferior MI. The size of inferior MI is proportional to the sum of ST elevation in the three inferior leads. In addition, those with reciprocal ST depression in anterior or lateral leads tend to have larger infarctions. Using these criteria, patient A was having the largest MI, patients B and C, moderate-sized MIs, and patient D, a small infarct. Patient B also had ST elevation in V₅ and V₆; this may be called an inferolateral MI. In this case, the distal right coronary artery in the AV groove was large, and it terminated in a branch to the lateral wall (see Fig 2.8).

   Patient D is an arguable case of infarction, as the ST segment elevation is minimal. I am tempted to say that the mild J-point depression in V₂ through V₄ represents reciprocal ST depression; typical chest pain and a subsequent rise in cardiac enzymes would be needed to make the diagnosis of MI with certainty in this case. The ECG changes of transmural infarction are usually obvious, but there are borderline cases like this one. As a rule, such borderline cases involve small MI's; big ones are obvious.

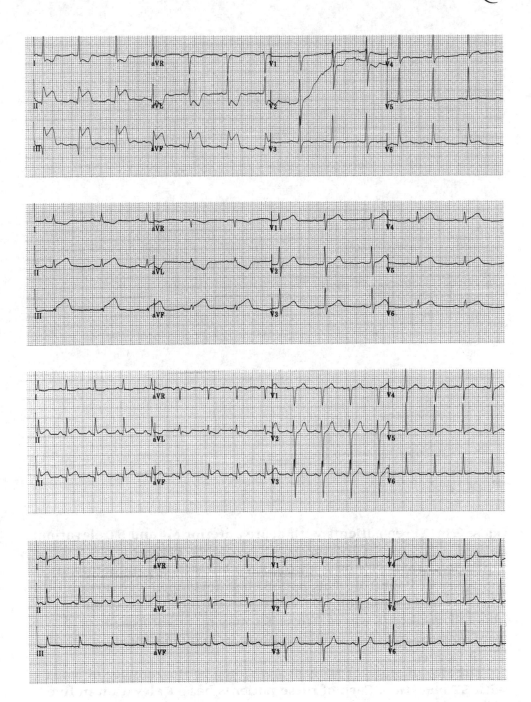

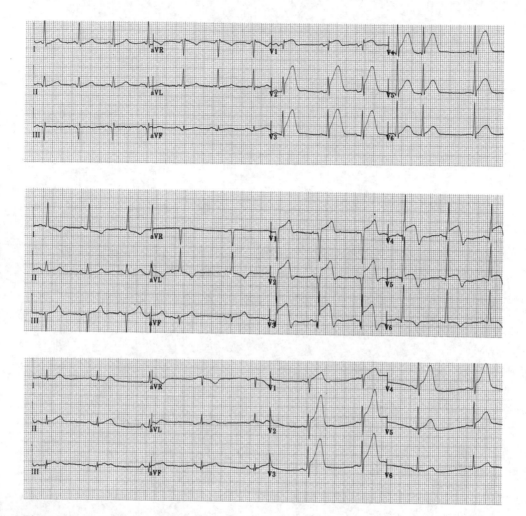

Figure 2.14 Three patients with acute anterior MI and ST elevation. Patient A has upwardly convex ST segments. Patient B has similarly shaped ST's in V$_3$ through V$_5$, but still has some upward concavity in V$_1$ and V$_2$. This patient has developed T inversion in addition to ST elevation (see Table 2.3). Patient C has ST elevation plus tall, peaked T waves. These T's may be called *hyperacute T wave changes,* and they would indicate ischemia in the absence of ST elevation.

The size of anterior MI is proportional to the number of leads with ST elevation. Each of these patients has ST elevation in five different leads and is having large infarction.

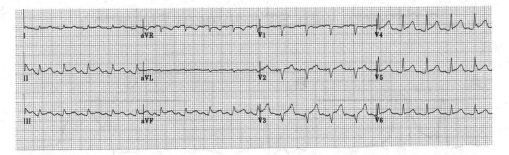

Figure 2.15 Acute pericarditis. This 19-year-old man had a 2-week history of the flu. There was mild fever. On the morning of this ECG, he developed chest pain that worsened with deep breathing (i.e., pleurisy). On exam, there was a pericardial friction rub. The ECG shows ST elevation in multiple leads, and there is no reciprocal ST depression. The ST's are upwardly concave. I think there is depression of the PR segment in lead II and aVF, an admittedly subtle finding.

ited to leads that reflect a single vascular distribution (see Fig 2.8). Patients with large transmural infarction who have ST segment elevation may also have ST depression in leads reflecting nonischemic myocardial regions (see Fig 2.13). The ST depression is called **reciprocal ST depression,** and it does not indicate ischemia in the noninfarct zone.

Although more reliable than ST segment depression, ST elevation is not specific for ischemia, and it must be interpreted in clinical context. Two non-ischemic causes of ST elevation deserve special attention.

1. Acute pericarditis may cause ST elevation and chest pain, raising the possibility of acute MI (Figs 2.15, 2.16). Features that may help you distinguish the ST elevation of pericarditis from that caused by ischemia are reviewed in Table 2.4. Although these features are helpful when found, they may also be subtle or missing. There is often uncertainty about the diagnosis, and the ECG is just one piece of the puzzle. The clinical presentation is just as important as the ECG.

2. Early repolarization is a frequent cause of ST elevation. The cause is not certain, but the name suggests that some portion of the ventricle repolarizes before the obvious onset of the T wave, raising the ST segment. As with pericarditis, the ST segment elevation may be global rather than regional (although it may be limited to just one or two leads), and the ST segment usually has normal upward concavity. It is often difficult to distinguish early repolarization and acute pericarditis. Early repolarization is a benign condition, common in young people. There is little day-to-day variation in this pattern, so comparison of the ECG with previous tracings should help make the diagnosis.

3 Patients with ST Segment Elevation

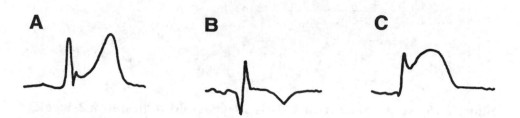

A   **B**   **C**

Figure 2.16 ST segment elevation. Patient A still has the normal upward concavity of the ST segment. This is usually the case with pericarditis, although we have seen similar ST changes with acute, transmural ischemia (see Fig 2.14). Patient B has simultaneous ST elevation and T inversion. This combination is a good indicator of ischemia. The T waves may invert with pericarditis, but the ST's usually become isoelectric before the T's turn over. Patient C has an upwardly convex ST segment; this usually indicates ischemia.

Q Waves and Evolution of Myocardial Infarction

An initial negative deflection of the QRS complex is labeled a Q wave. A significant Q wave is deep and broad (1 mm deep and 1 mm wide). Isolated Q waves may be found in either III or V_1; in other leads, Q waves are abnormal and indicate transmural myocardial injury.

In the absence of acute reperfusion therapy, the ECG pattern of MI evolves over a couple of days (Fig 2.17 and Table 2.3). The earliest change

Table 2.4 ST Segment Elevation: Pericarditis versus Ischemia

	PERICARDITIS	ISCHEMIA
Distribution	Global (multiple vascular distributions)	Regional (one vascular distribution)
Reciprocal ST depression	Absent	May be present
ST segment shape	Normal (upwardly concave)	Ischemic (upwardly convex)
PR depression	Present (see Fig 2.15)	Absent
Timing of T inversion	T's invert after ST's become isoelectric	T's invert while the ST's are still elevated

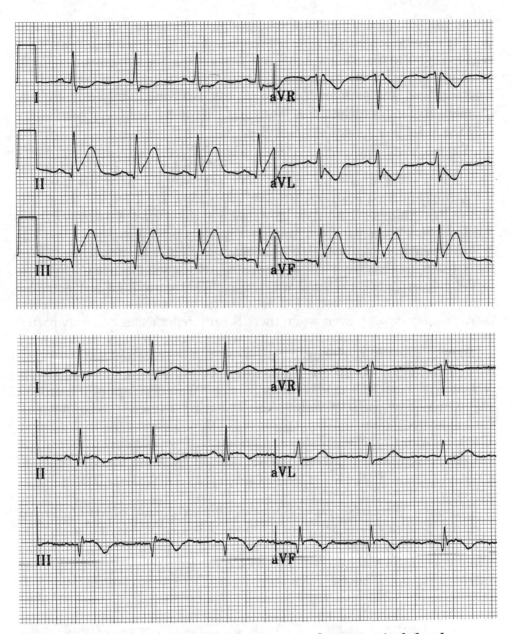

Figure 2.17 Typical evolution of transmural MI. A: Limb leads from a patient with acute MI who had inferior ST elevation plus reciprocal ST depression in lateral leads. B: The next day there was less ST elevation, the reciprocal ST depression had resolved, and the T waves were inverted in the inferior leads. Deeper Q waves developed in the inferior leads.

is ST segment elevation, and this develops immediately with coronary occlusion. It may be associated with tall, peaked T waves called **hyperacute T waves** (Fig 2.14D). Within hours, the T waves may become inverted while there is persistence of ST elevation. Hours to days after the onset of MI, Q waves appear. The diagnosis of MI is most secure when these evolutionary changes are recorded by serial ECGs. ST elevation without evolutionary changes suggests a nonischemic etiology.

While ST elevation and T wave inversion may resolve during the 2 weeks after acute MI, Q waves persist in 70% to 90% of patients. They may disappear after a small inferior MI, but Q's tend to be permanent after a large MI.

Acute **reperfusion therapy** for MI has changed some of this. The evolution of ECG changes is more rapid. As soon as the occluded infarct artery is opened, the ST segment elevation either resolves or improves. Q waves develop rapidly with reperfusion, possibly within minutes. Our experience with reperfusion also has provided new insights into the significance of Q waves. In the old days, I was taught that Q waves meant transmural scar with loss of all muscle (and, therefore, a loss of contractility). Now we know that deep Q waves may develop even when there is early reperfusion and only partial injury to muscle in the infarct zone. Q waves do not reliably define an LV segment as irreversibly damaged—or the infarction as completed.

The concept of **complete vs. incomplete MI** is important clinically. A patient who has had a Q wave infarction but who develops postinfarction angina may have viable muscle in the infarct zone (the source of angina). The usual mechanism for this is spontaneous thrombolysis early in the course of MI. As with thrombolytic therapy, an hour or two of ischemia is enough to cause Q waves, even though injury is incomplete and there is residual, viable muscle. In fact, early reperfusion seems to hasten the evolution of Q waves.

This same mechanism may be at work with **extension of MI.** Recurrent pain, more ST elevation, and another increase in cardiac enzyme during the week after a Q wave infarction may indicate that the initial infarction was incomplete, possibly because of spontaneous thrombolysis. Reocclusion of the infarct artery is responsible for recurrence, or "extension," of the MI.

Lateral Wall MI

By ECG criteria, transmural MI is defined by pathologic Q waves. Occlusion of the circumflex artery may cause ST segment elevation in lateral leads (Figs 2.8, 2.18). However, it is possible to have transmural injury involving the lateral wall of the LV with few ST segment or T wave changes and without Q waves. The lateral wall seems to be an electrocardiographically silent region of the heart (see Fig 2.8). The patient may have typical chest pain and a subse-

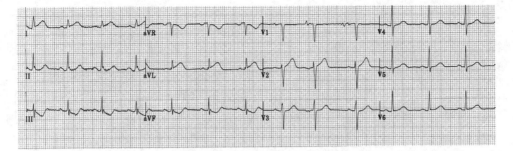

Figure 2.18 Acute lateral MI. ST elevation is limited to the lateral leads, I, and aVL. It is possible to have ST changes in just V₆, or in V₅ and V₆. And it is also possible to have lateral, transmural ischemia with no ECG changes at all.

quent rise in cardiac enzymes and may even be left with akinesis (no contractility) of the lateral wall. Yet he or she may have a normal ECG throughout the course of MI. This is the rationale for admitting a person with typical, ischemic chest pain but a normal ECG to the hospital for overnight observation.

Silent MI, Pseudo MI

The opposite side of the coin is the patient with no symptoms who has significant Q waves and an akinetic LV segment involving the same vascular region (i.e., anterior Q waves and anterior akinesis on the echocardiogram). Taking a careful history, you could get the patient to remember vague symptoms that could have been the infarction, but in many cases there are no symptoms at all. This is the case with at least 10% of MI's, and it may be more common in patients with diabetes and diabetic neuropathy.

On occasion, Q waves are seen with LVH or other conditions that cause PRWP (false positive Q waves, or a pseudoinfarction pattern). When there are unexplained Q waves, the possibility of silent MI must be considered. A good first step is an echocardiogram or radionuclide angiogram looking for an LV regional wall motion abnormality. It is important to recognize silent ischemic heart disease, because it is associated with poor prognosis.

A couple of conditions may produce false positive Q waves. The delta wave of pre-excitation may appear to be a Q wave (Fig 2.19). Recognition of the short PR interval, the absence of a clinical history of MI, and a normal echocardiogram are tipoffs. Q waves may be seen in patients with hypertrophic cardiomyopathy, and the diagnosis is made by an echocardiogram.

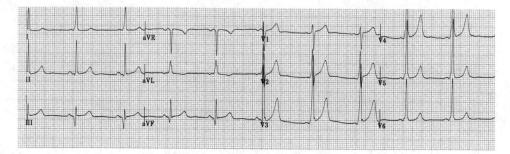

Figure 2.19 Pseudoinfarction pattern caused by pre-excitation (WPW). The inferior Q's are, in fact, delta waves. The tipoff is the short PR interval plus the more obvious delta wave in the lateral precordial leads.

Drugs and Metabolic Abnormalities That May Alter the ECG and Cardiac Rhythm

Table 1.2 (pps. 11–12) summarizes conditions and drugs that may alter intervals and ECG morphology. Table 2.5 completes this summary, reviewing changes in rate and rhythm. I have tried to cover conditions and drugs that you will encounter most frequently while reading routine ECGs (and taking Board exams).

Table 2.5 ECG Abnormalities Caused by Drugs and Metabolic Conditions

	DRUGS	METABOLIC CONDITIONS
Rate		
Sinus bradycardia	Beta adrenergic blockers, calcium blockers (verapamil and diltiazem), digitalis, intravenous adenosine	Hypoxemia, hypothyroidism, hyperkalemia, hypothermia
Sinus tachycardia	Catecholamines, caffeine, amphetamines	Hyperthyroidism, anemia, fever
Rhythm		
Heart block	Digitalis, beta adrenergic blockers, calcium blockers (verapamil, diltiazem), intravenous adenosine	Hyperkalemia
Atrial flutter		Hypoxemia (consider pulmonary embolus)
Atrial fibrillation	Thyroid hormone	Hyperthyroidism
Ventricular tachycardia/fibrillation	Most antiarrhythmic agents (proarrhythmia), digoxin, tricyclic overdose	Hypokalemia, hypomagnesemia, hypocalcemia
Torsade de pointe	Class I (antiarrhythmic agents (quinidine, procainamide, disopyramide), sotalol, amiodarone, phenothiazine derivatives (including antihistamines), tricyclic overdose	Long QT syndrome

II

150

Practice

ECGs

As you read the practice ECGs, write the ECG report including rate, rhythm, intervals, axis, and interpretation. If you do not commit yourself on paper, it does not count! Read five to ten ECGs in a row before checking answers. There is a rhythm to this exercise that you should not interrupt. By the end of the section, you will be much more confident in your ability. Then go back and re-read the earlier ECGs—they will seem like unknowns.

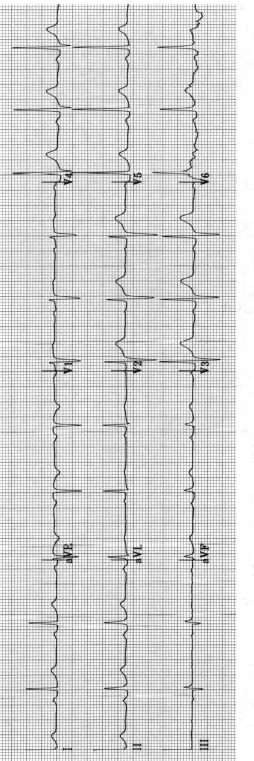

Practice ECG 1 57 year-old man, preoperative ECG.

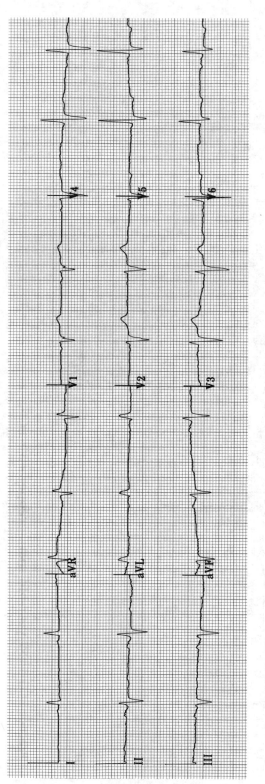

Practice ECG 2   78 year-old man, no history provided.

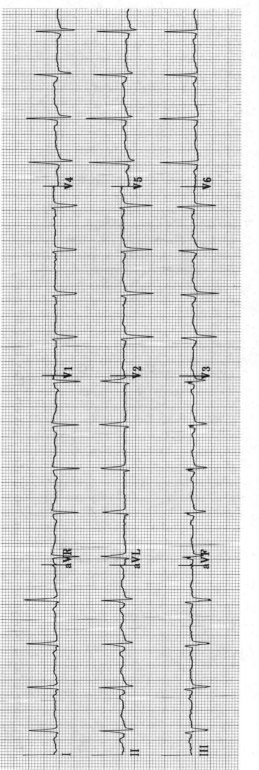

Practice ECG 3 54 year-old woman, admitted with cholecystitis.

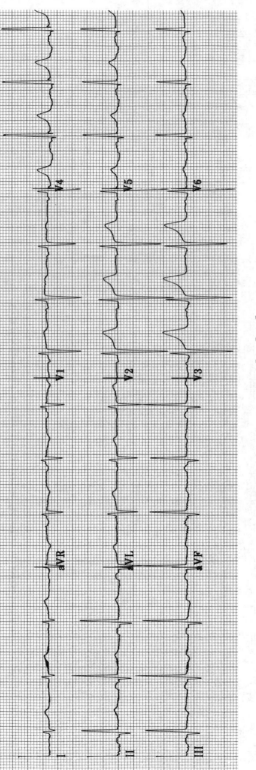

Practice ECG 4   49 year-old man, no history given. Has he had an MI? When?

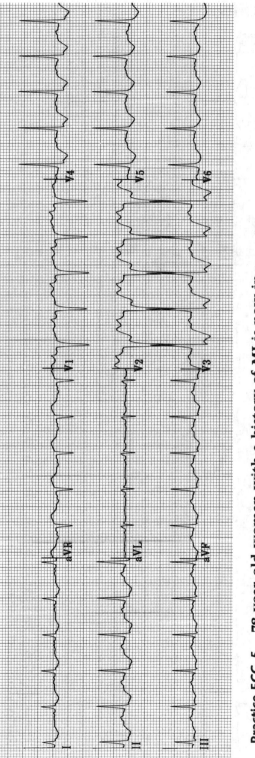
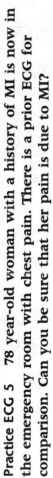

Practice ECG 5   **78 year-old woman with a history of MI is now in the emergency room with chest pain. There is a prior ECG for comparison. Can you be sure that her pain is due to MI?**

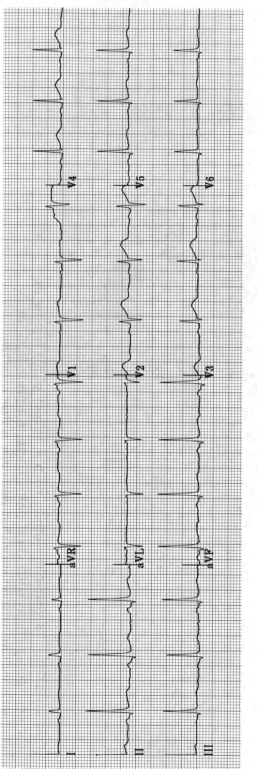

Practice ECG 6   36 year-old man; life insurance examination, no history of heart disease.

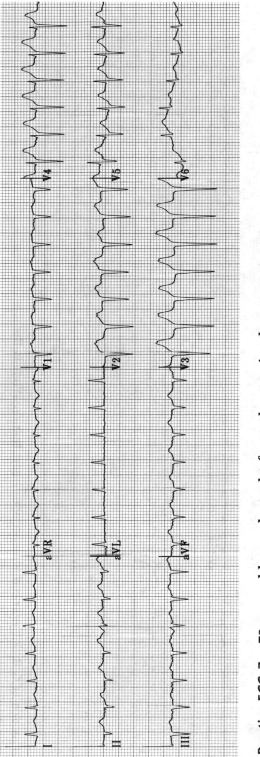

Practice ECG 7   79 year-old man brought from the nursing home with a rapid pulse.

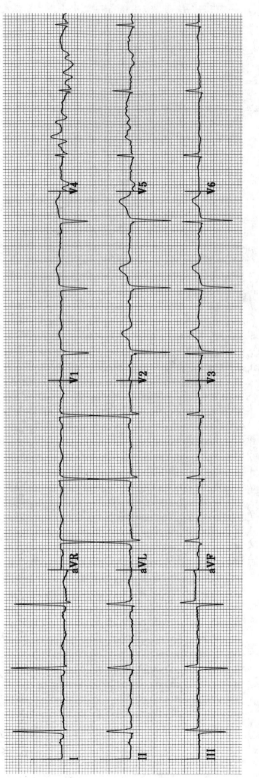

Practice ECG 8 72 year-old woman with heart failure. What is the etiology?

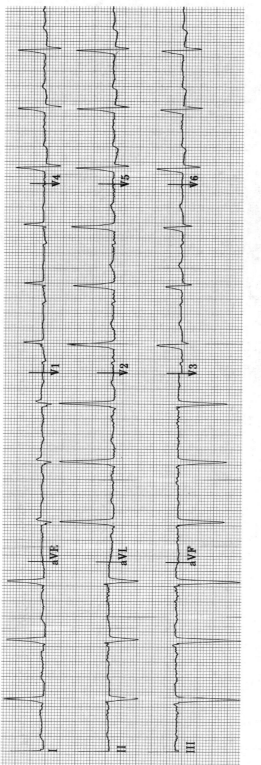
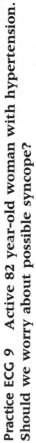

Practice ECG 9   Active 82 year-old woman with hypertension. Should we worry about possible syncope?

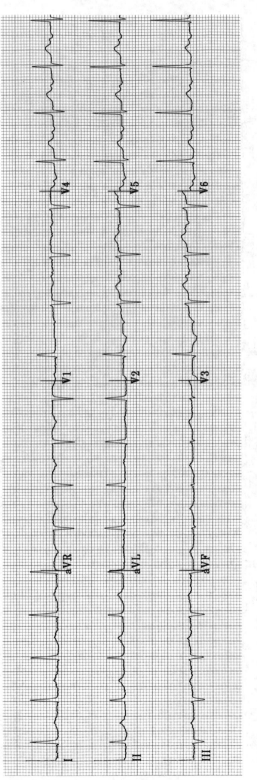

Practice ECG 10   94 year-old woman with failing memory.

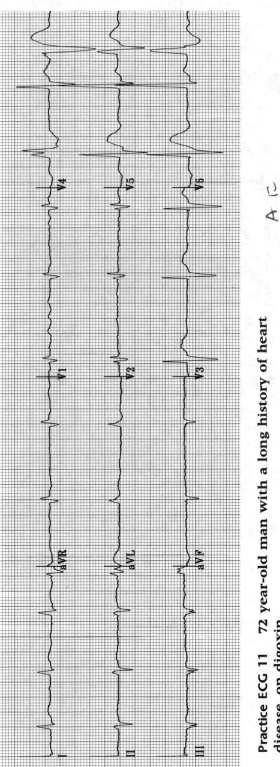

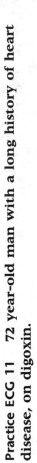

Practice ECG 11   72 year-old man with a long history of heart disease, on digoxin.

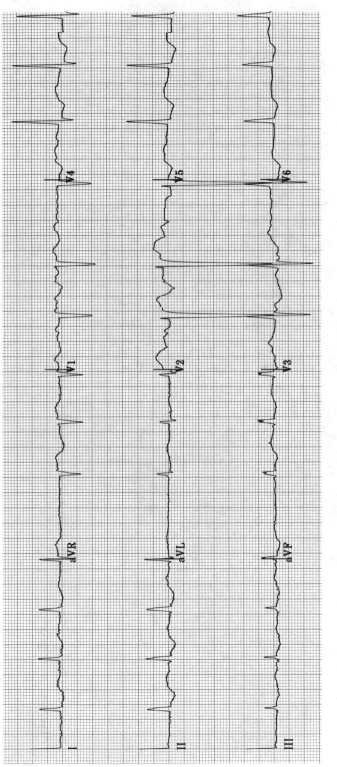

Practice ECG 12   73 year-old woman with hypertension, on multiple medicines. Can you identify one of them?

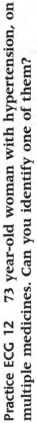

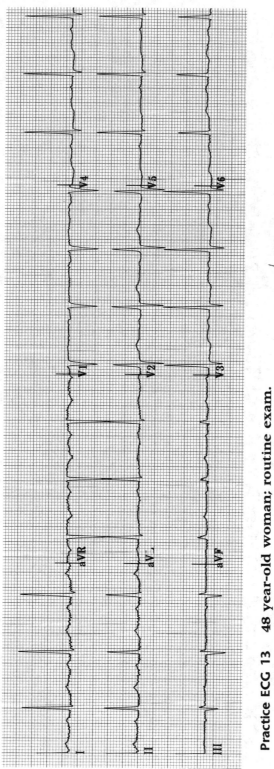
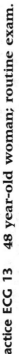

Practice ECG 13   48 year-old woman; routine exam.

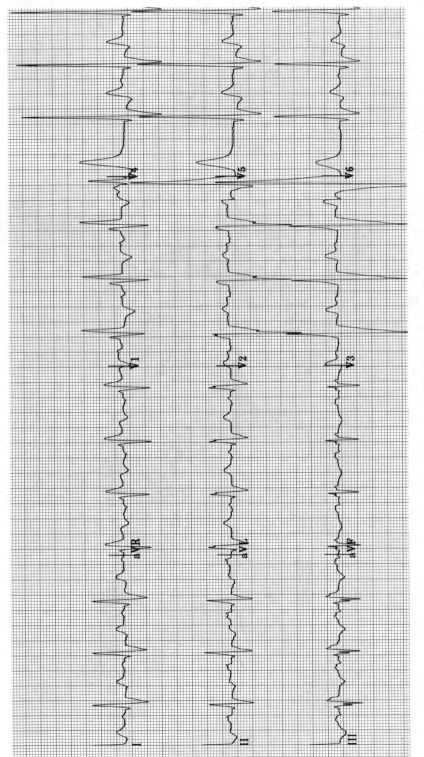
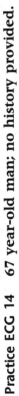

Practice ECG 14   67 year-old man; no history provided.

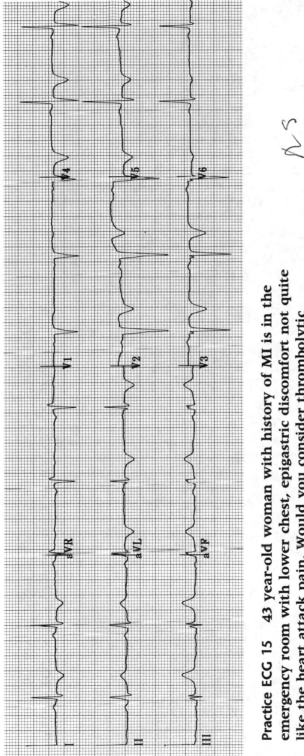

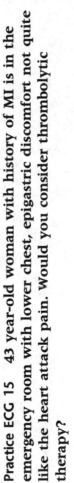

Practice ECG 15 **43 year-old woman with history of MI is in the emergency room with lower chest, epigastric discomfort not quite like the heart attack pain. Would you consider thrombolytic therapy?**

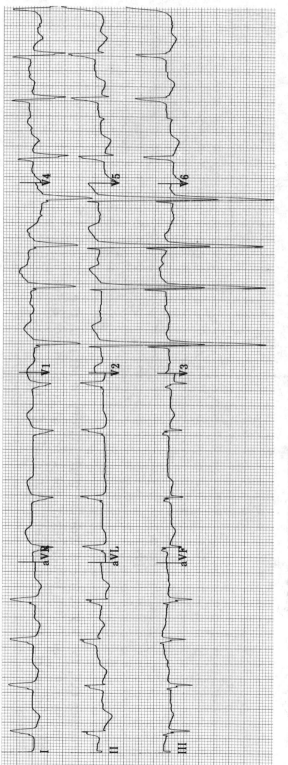

Practice ECG 16 73 year-old woman with blood pressure 170/75 and no history of heart disease. Should she be treated for

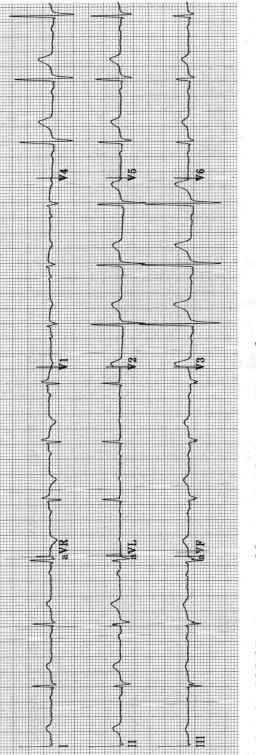

Practice ECG 17 46 year-old man; routine exam. Normal or abnormal?

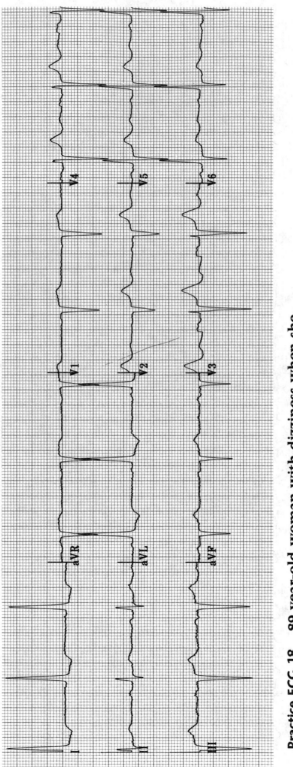

Practice ECG 18   89 year-old woman with dizziness when she stands.

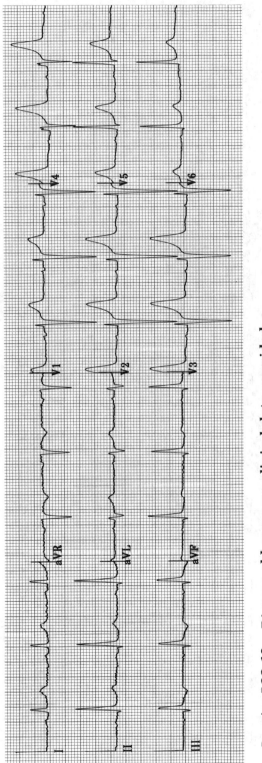

Practice ECG 19   74 year-old man; no clinical data provided.

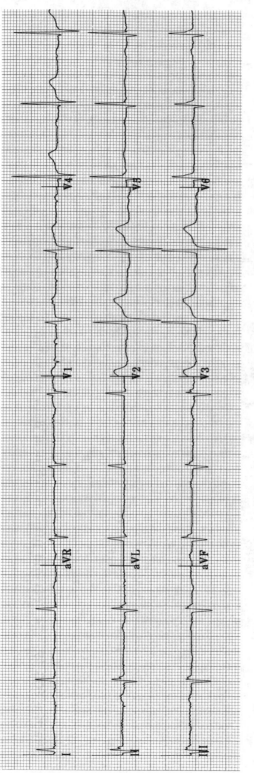

Practice ECG 20   76 year-old man with history of MI and mild heart failure. Does this ECG tell you anything about the patient's coronary anatomy?

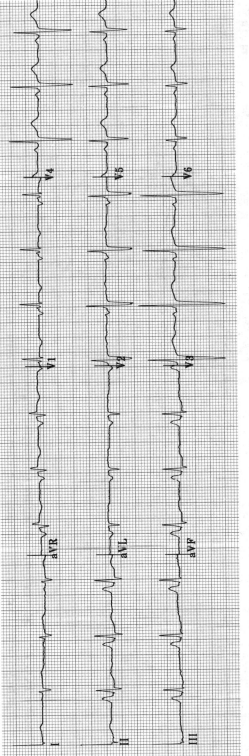
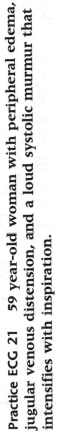

Practice ECG 21   59 year-old woman with peripheral edema, jugular venous distension, and a loud systolic murmur that intensifies with inspiration.

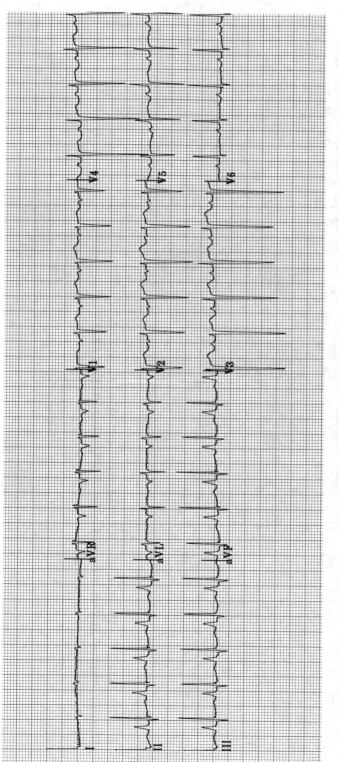

Practice ECG 22   56 year-old woman admitted through the emergency room. Any guess about the nature of her acute illness?

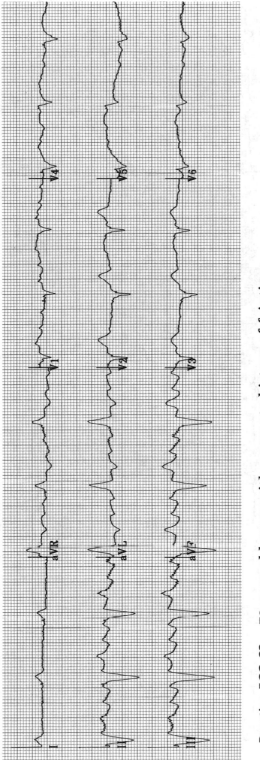

Practice ECG 23 70 year-old man with a remote history of fainting spells. Now in the emergency room with dyspnea and fever.

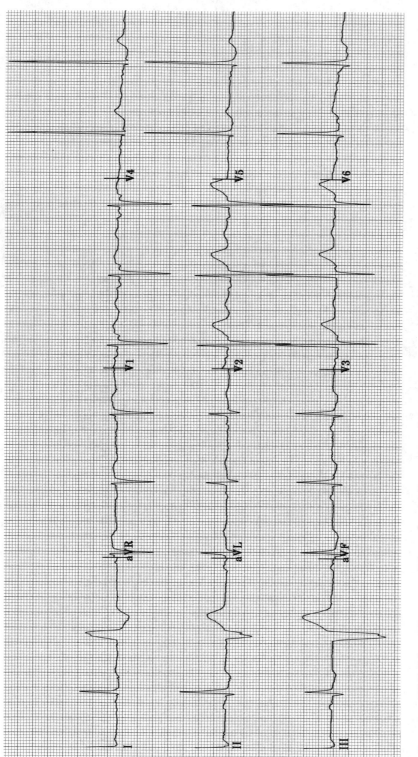

Practice ECG 24   75 year-old man with a systolic murmur and heart failure. What is the dominant valvular lesion?

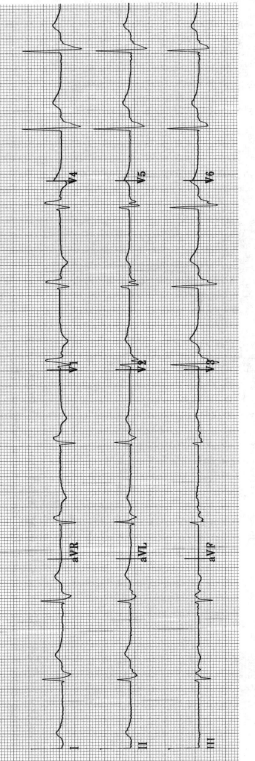

Practice ECG 25 **80 year-old man treated with diuretics and digoxin. What lab work is needed?**

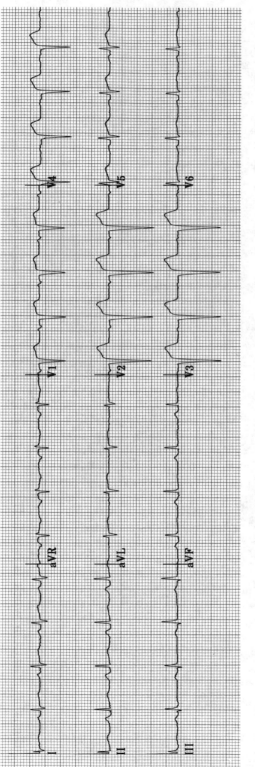

Practice ECG 26 52 year-old man who had a 20-hour siege of indigestion a month earlier. He has severe fatigue. The cardiologist has ordered an echocardiogram. Why?

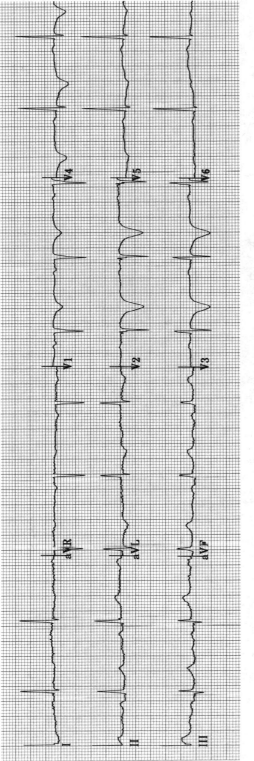

Practice ECG 27   71 year-old woman in the emergency room. A long episode of chest pain was relieved before her arrival by nitroglycerine. Is angiography indicated? What would it show?

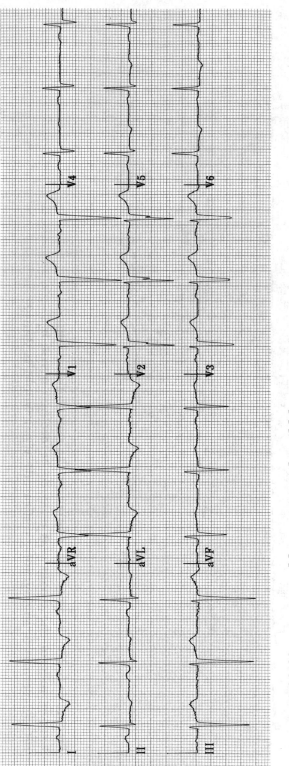

Practice ECG 28   79 year-old woman with mild hypertension.

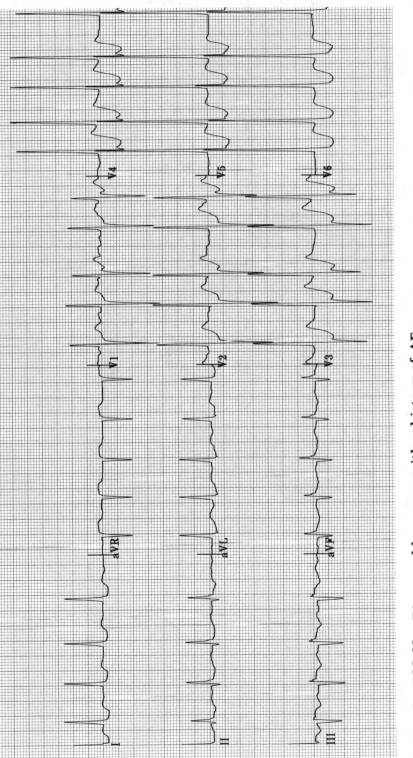

Practice ECG 29 74 year-old woman with a history of AF, diabetes, hypertension, obesity, and MI. Now in the emergency room with pulmonary edema.

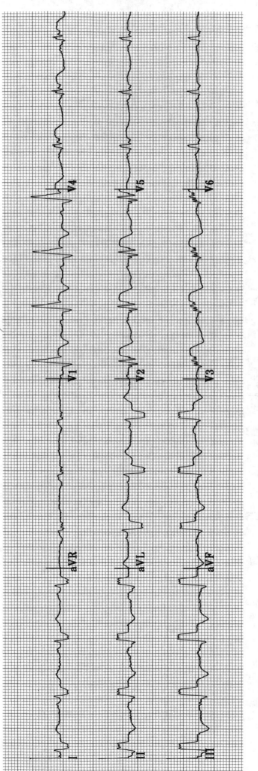
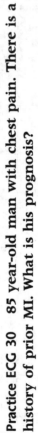

Practice ECG 30 85 year-old man with chest pain. There is a history of prior MI. What is his prognosis?

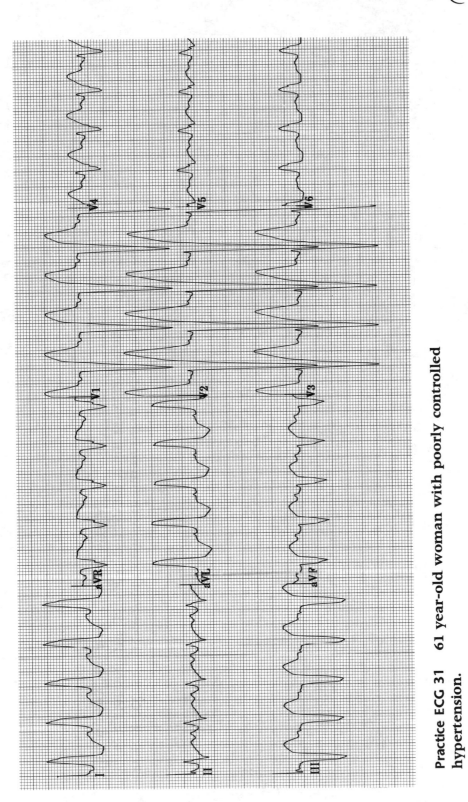

Practice ECG 31   61 year-old woman with poorly controlled hypertension.

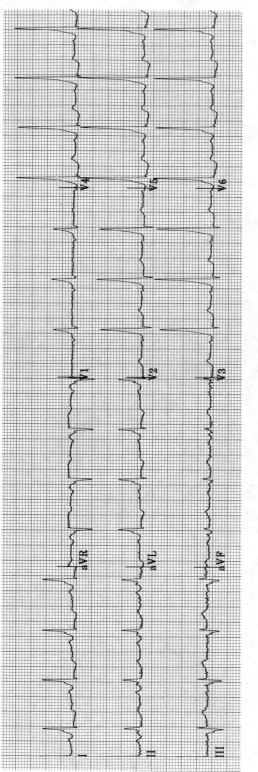
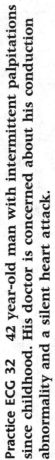

Practice ECG 32   42 year-old man with intermittent palpitations since childhood. His doctor is concerned about his conduction abnormality and a silent heart attack.

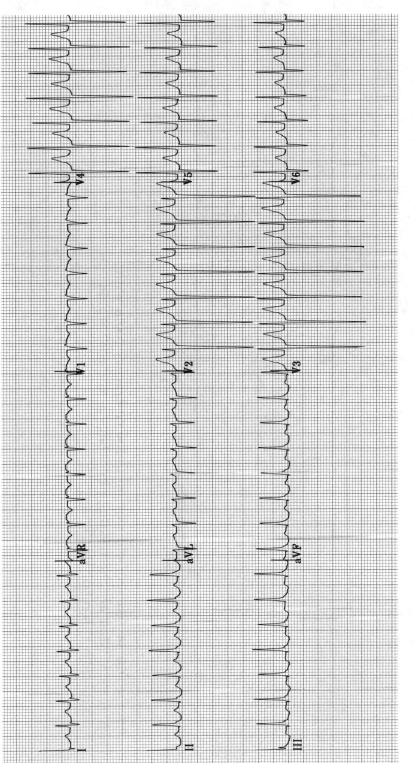

Practice ECG 33 38 year-old woman with palpitations and dizziness.

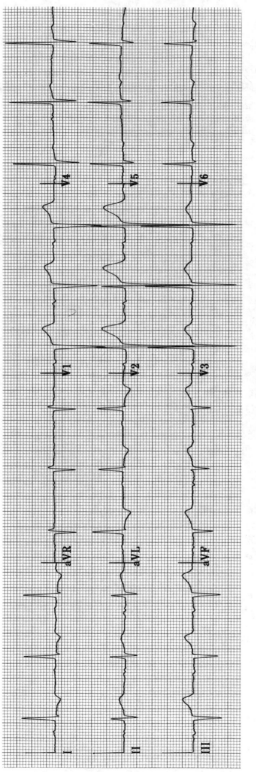

Practice ECG 34 · 81 year-old woman in the emergency room with chest pain. What are the treating physician's next steps? Would you consider thrombolytic therapy?

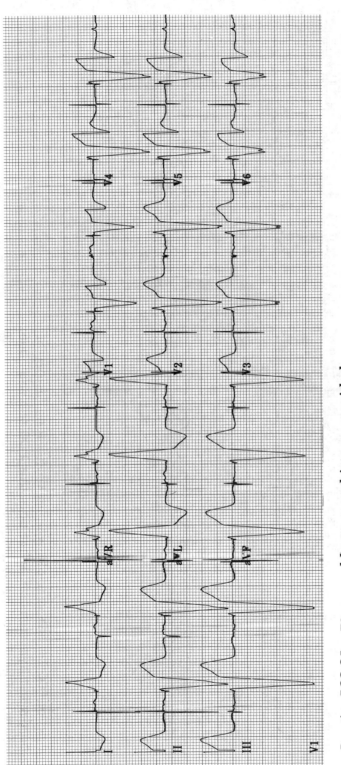

Practice ECG 35   73 year-old man; no history provided.

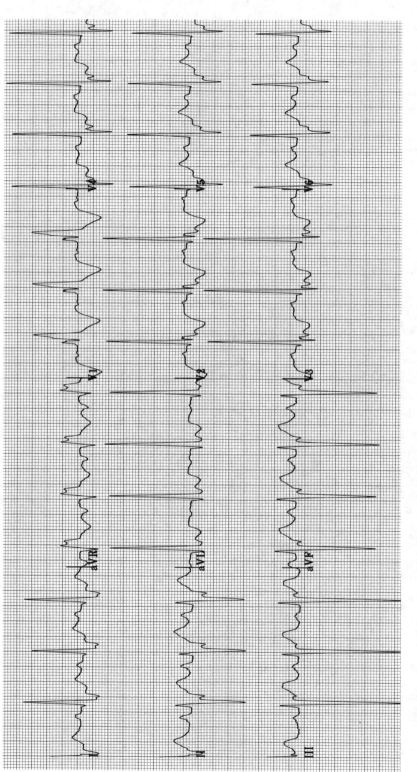

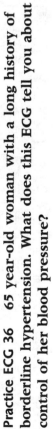

Practice ECG 36   65 year-old woman with a long history of borderline hypertension. What does this ECG tell you about control of her blood pressure?

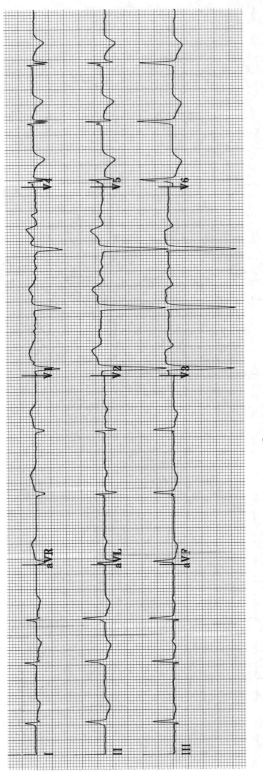

Practice ECG 37   86 year-old woman, annual ECG.

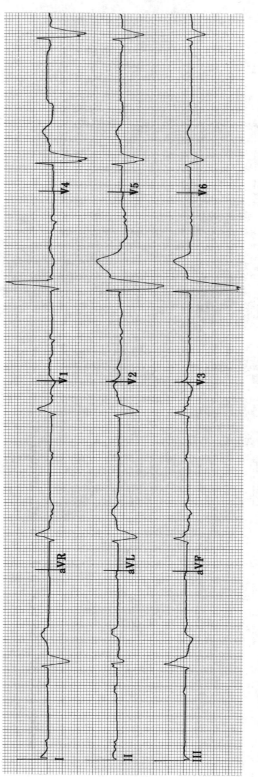

Practice ECG 38   82 year-old man with fatigue and ankle edema for 2 weeks.

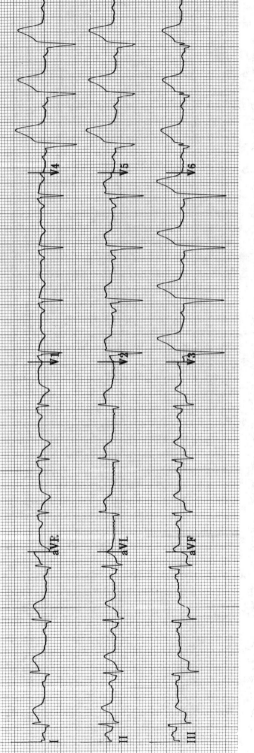

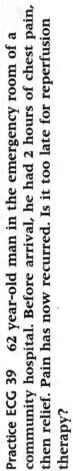

Practice ECG 39 62 year-old man in the emergency room of a community hospital. Before arrival, he had 2 hours of chest pain, then relief. Pain has now recurred. Is it too late for reperfusion therapy?

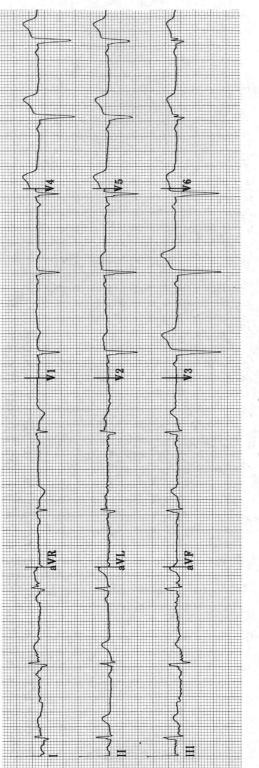

Practice ECG 40   Same patient (No. 39), 2 hours after treatment with tissue plasminogen activator.

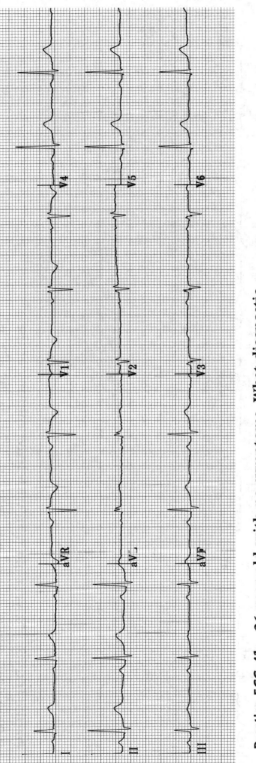

Practice ECG 41   26 year-old with no symptoms. What diagnostic test is needed?

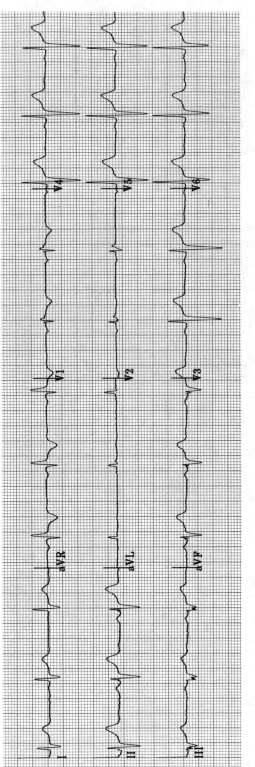

Practice ECG 42   32 year-old man with fixed splitting of the second heart sound and a loud murmur. What is the illness?

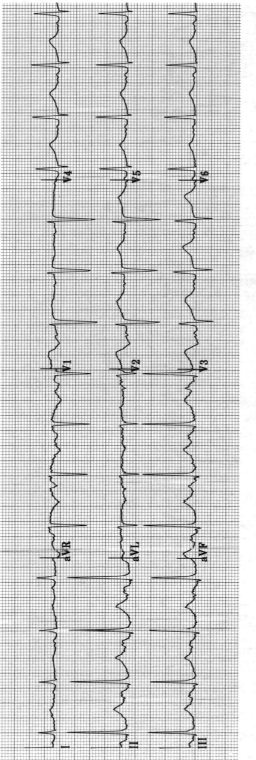
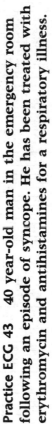

Practice ECG 43   40 year-old man in the emergency room following an episode of syncope. He has been treated with erythromycin and antihistamines for a respiratory illness.

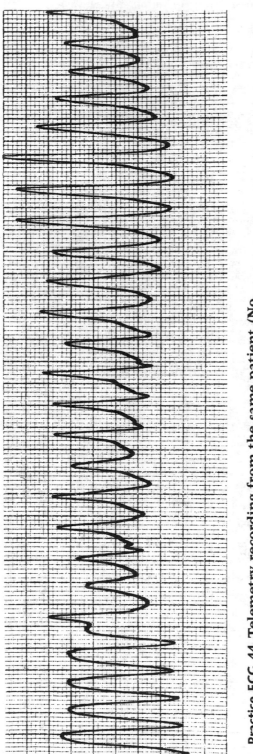

Practice ECG 44 Telemetry recording from the same patient (No. 43) 4 hours later. During the arrhythmia, he lost consciousness.

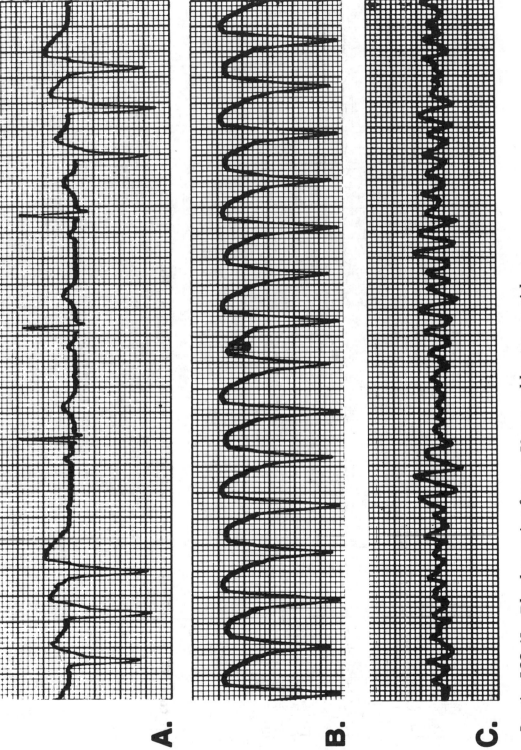

A.

B.

C.

Practice ECG 45   Rhythm strips from a 52 year-old woman with cardiomyopathy and episodic dizziness. During the third tracing, she lost consciousness.

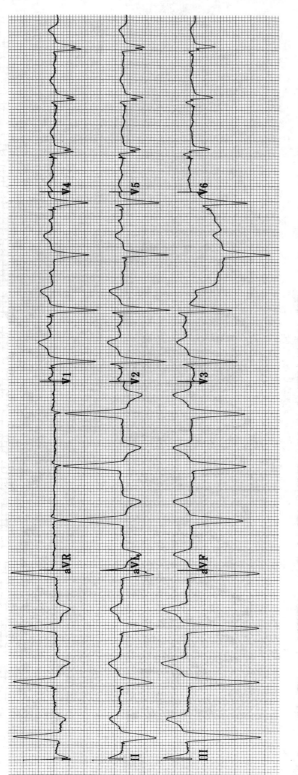
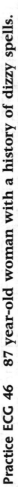

Practice ECG 46   87 year-old woman with a history of dizzy spells.

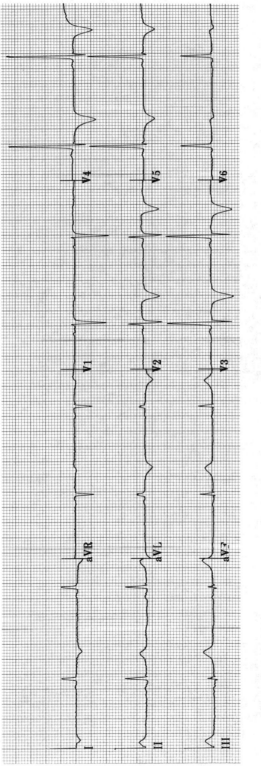

Practice ECG 47   **45 year-old man after a 45-minute episode of chest pain.**

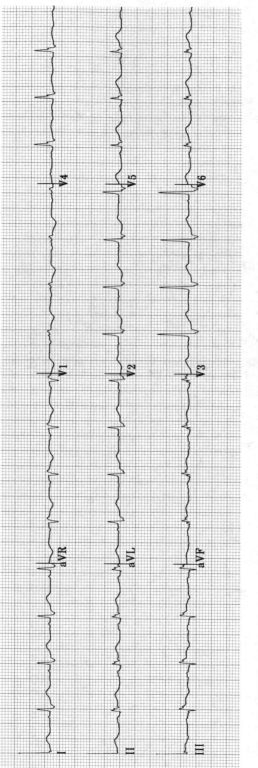

Practice ECG 48 68 year-old woman after 9 hours of indigestion. What treatment is indicated?

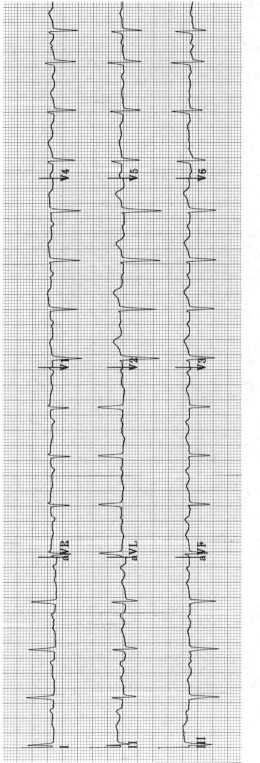

Practice ECG 49   76 year-old woman with diabetes; yearly examination.

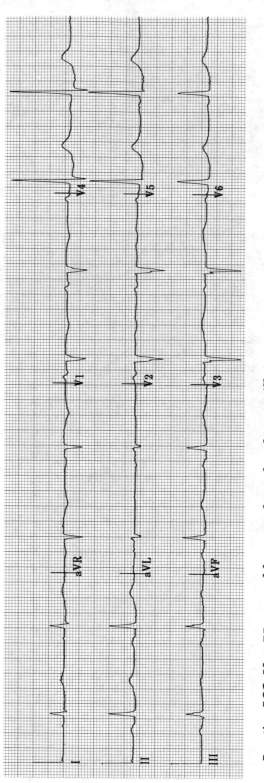

Practice ECG 50   75 year-old man who takes heart pills.

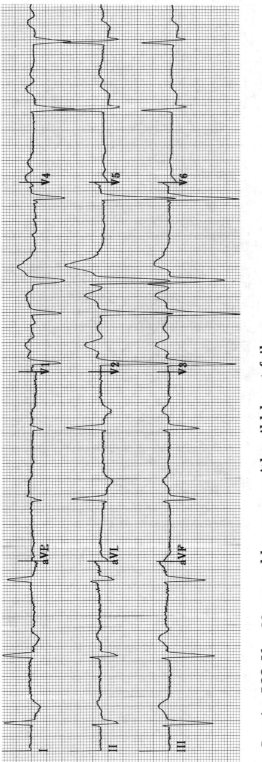

Practice ECG 51   82 year-old woman with mild heart failure.

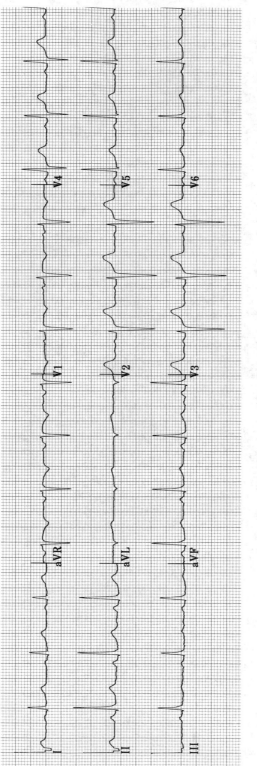

Practice ECG 52   53 year-old woman with hypertension and obesity, taking diuretics.

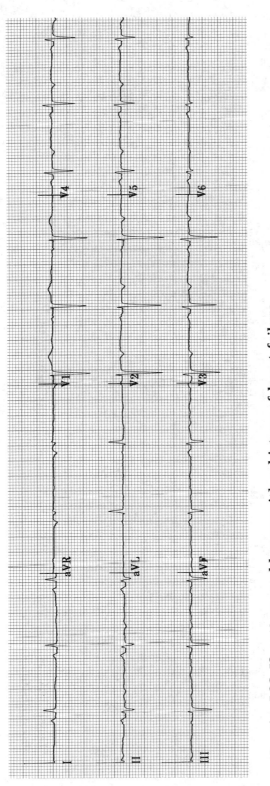

Practice ECG 53   69 year-old man with a history of heart failure.

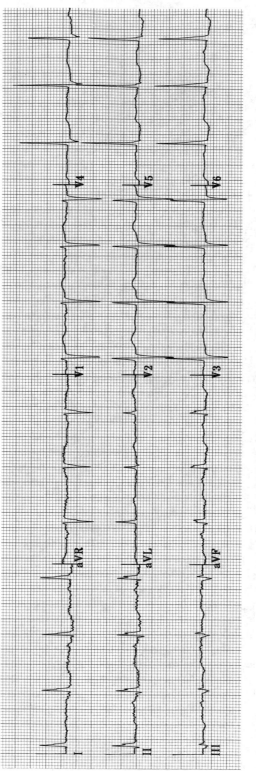

Practice ECG 54   70 year-old woman with a remote history of MI and a history of AF.

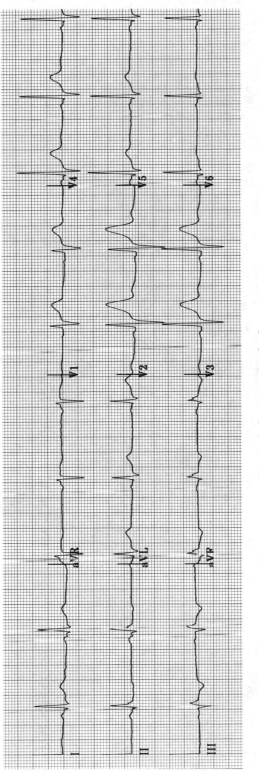

Practice ECG 55   60 year-old man; no clinical data provided.

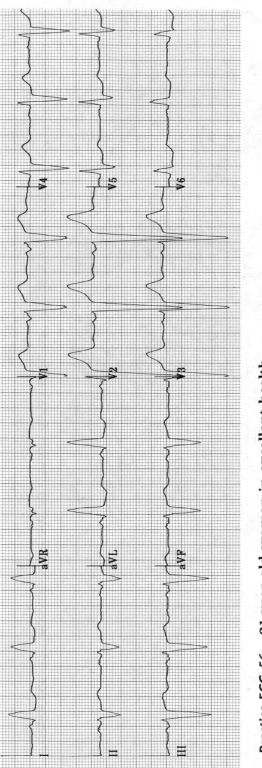

Practice ECG 56   81 year-old woman in excellent health.

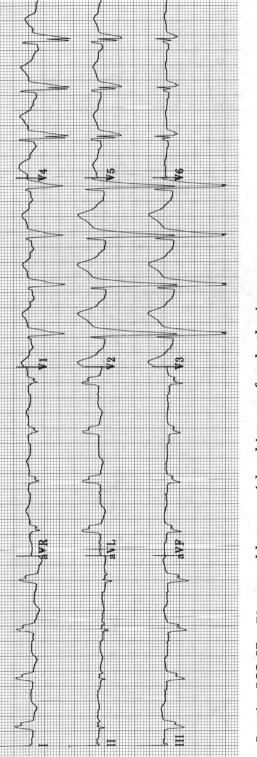

Practice ECG 57   72 year-old man with a history of arrhythmias.

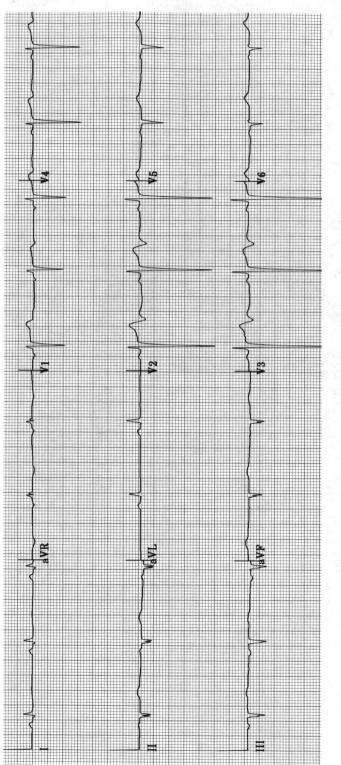

Practice ECG 58 31 year-old woman sent to a clinic because her ECG showed a heart attack. She had no history of MI. On exam there was a heart murmur.

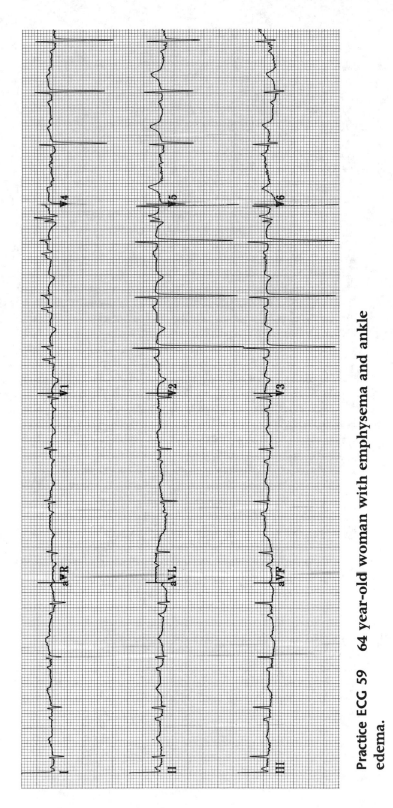

Practice ECG 59   64 year-old woman with emphysema and ankle edema.

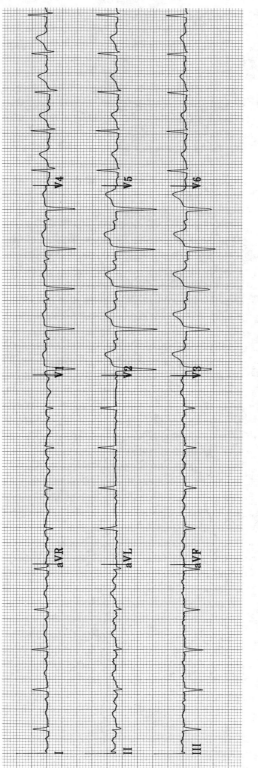

Practice ECG 60   79 year-old man with easy fatigue and exertional dyspnea.

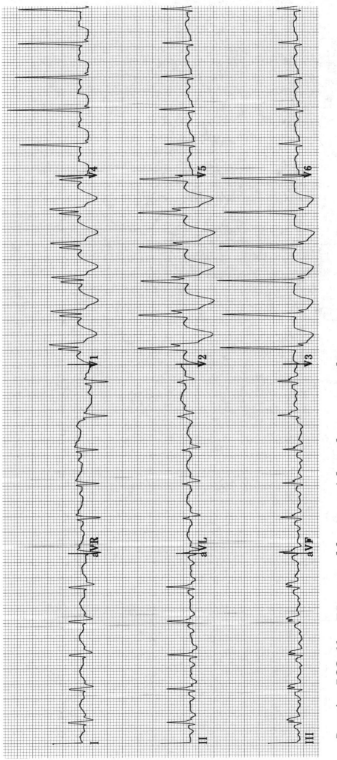

Practice ECG 61 75 year-old man with pulmonary edema.

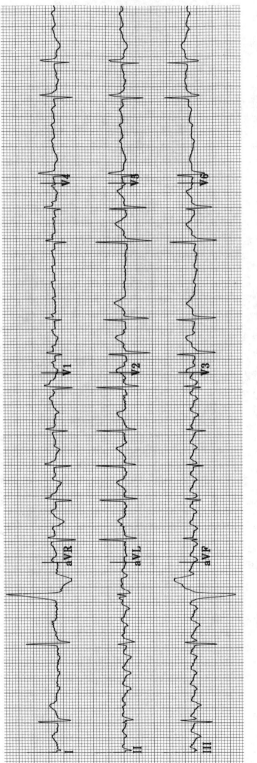

Practice ECG 62 83 year-old man with a long history of irregular pulse. He is on digoxin. Is another drug indicated?

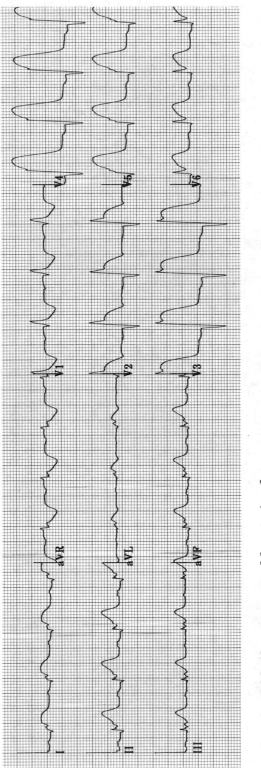

Practice ECG 63   59 year-old man in the emergency room.

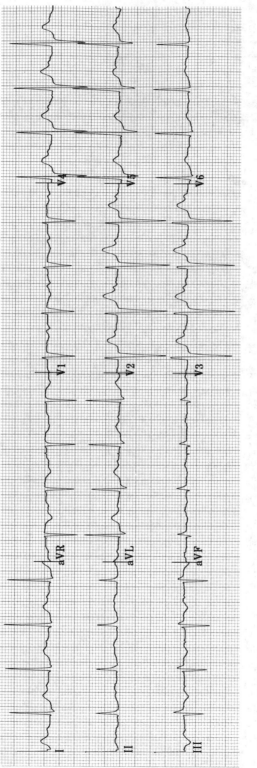

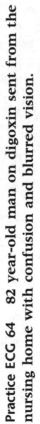

Practice ECG 64   82 year-old man on digoxin sent from the nursing home with confusion and blurred vision.

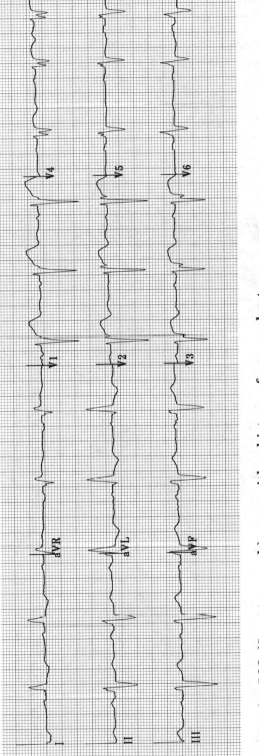

Practice ECG 65 66 year-old man with a history of vague chest pain and a positive stress test.

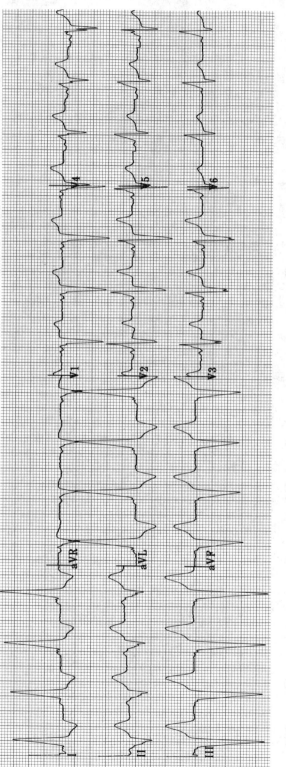

Practice ECG 66 26 year-old woman with palpitations. Her ECG was normal the day after this tracing was obtained.

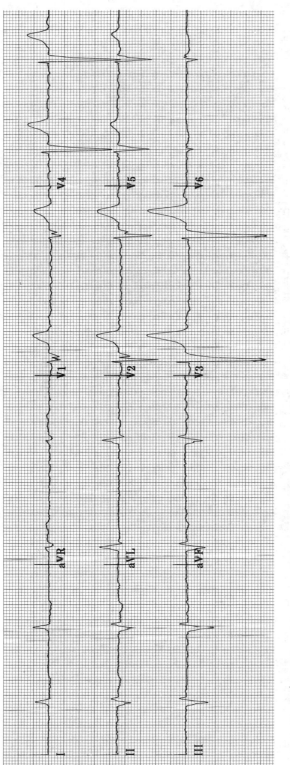

Practice ECG 67   86 year-old man with dizzy spells for 1 week, on no medicine. What should his doctor do?

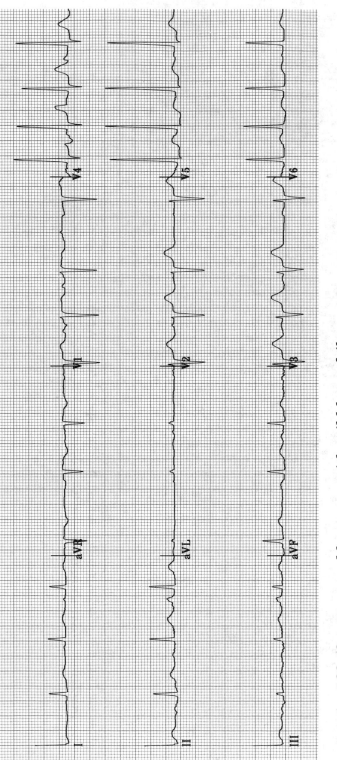

Practice ECG 68   85 year-old woman with mild heart failure, on digoxin.

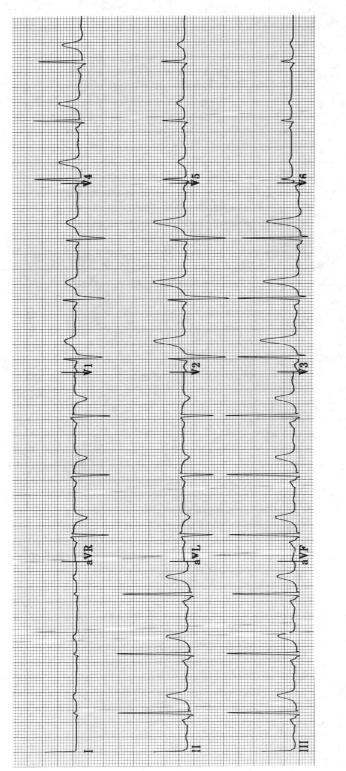

Practice ECG 69 70 year-old woman with ankle edema on two diuretics and potassium supplements.

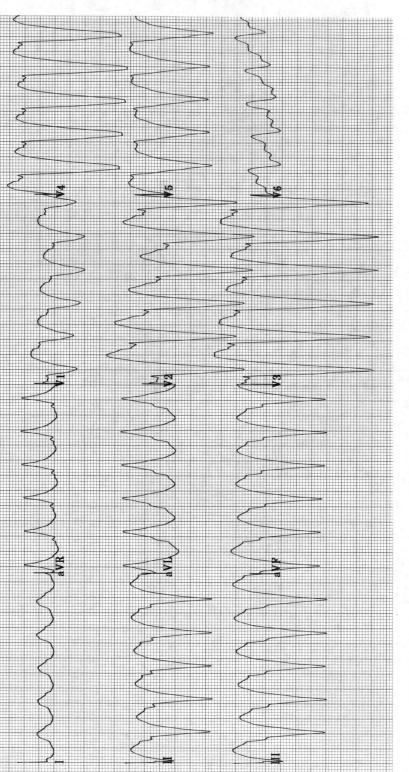

Practice ECG 70 77 year-old man in the emergency room with pounding in his chest.

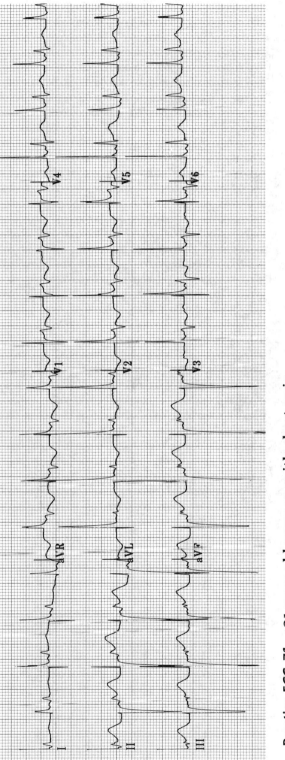

Practice ECG 71   81 year-old woman with chest pain.

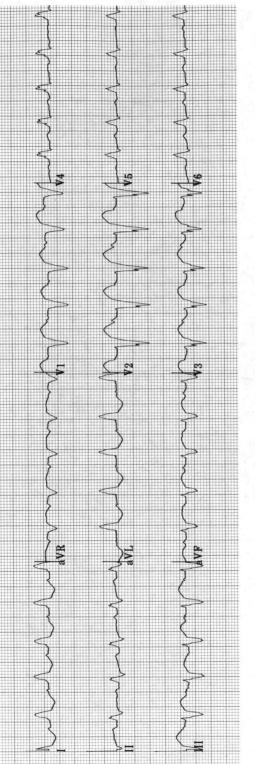

Practice ECG 72   78 year-old woman, postoperative ECG. The preoperative tracing showed mild IVCD.

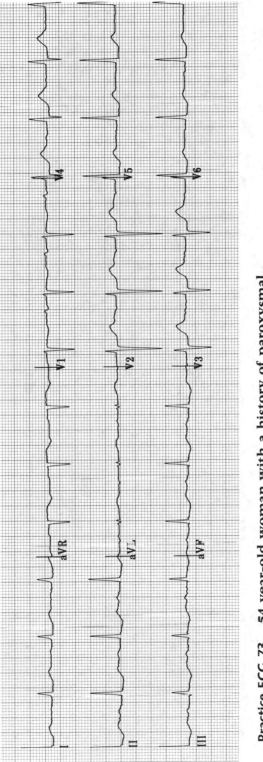

Practice ECG 73   54 year-old woman with a history of paroxysmal atrial fibrillation.

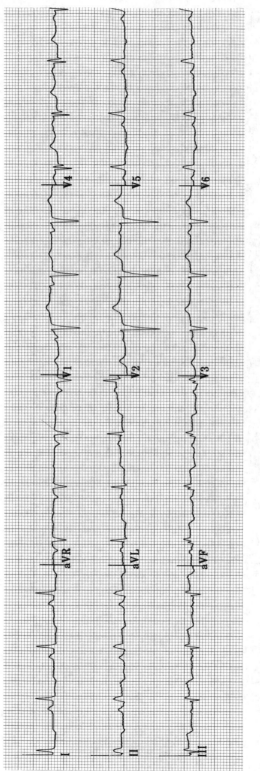

Practice ECG 74   72 year-old woman with chest pain for 2 hours. What is the correct treatment?

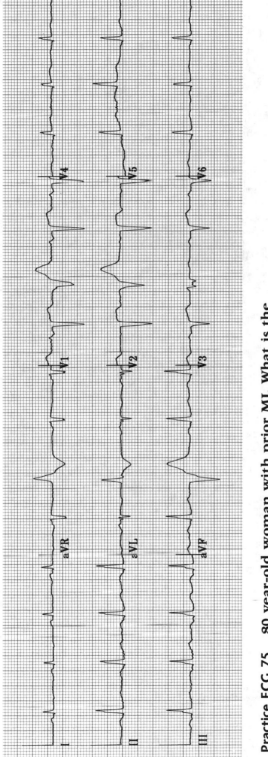

Practice ECG 75   80 year-old woman with prior MI. What is the origin of the ectopic beats?

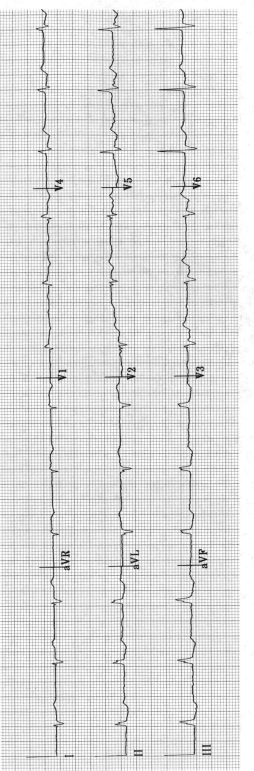

Practice ECG 76 64 year-old woman with chronic cough, dyspnea, and ankle edema. She still smokes two packs of cigarettes a day.

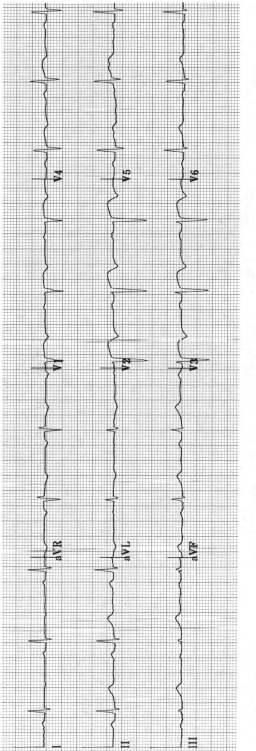

Practice ECG 77 67 year-old woman transferred because of a 1-hour episode of chest pain yesterday.

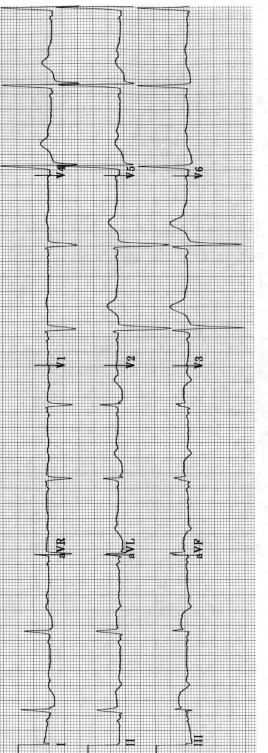

Figure 78 39 year-old farmer whose wife drove him to the local emergency room after 30 min of chest pain. He is 70 miles from the regional cardiac center. What is the correct treatment?

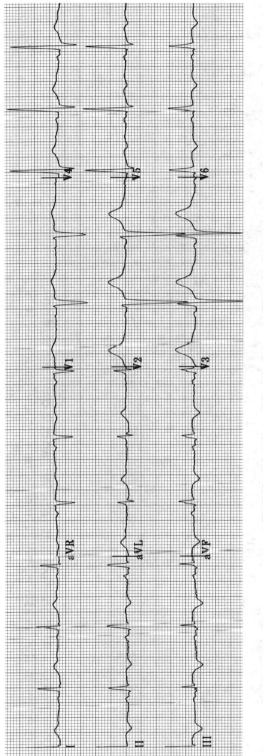

Practice ECG 79 Same patient (No. 78), about 1 hour later. Chest pain has resolved. What is the treatment now?

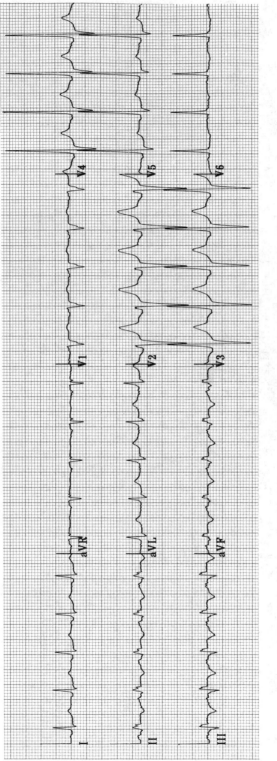

Practice ECG 80   Same patient (No. 78), after 2 days of heparin therapy in the local hospital. There is more chest pain, but it is not quite like what he had at the time of admission.

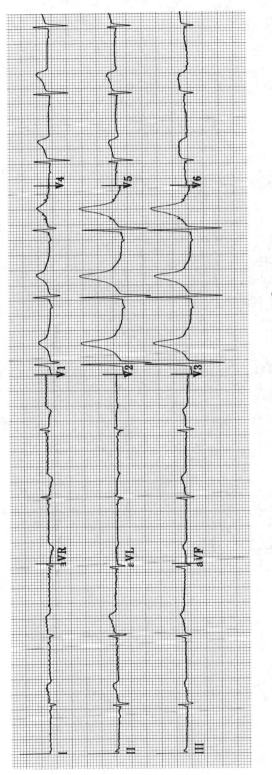

Practice ECG 81 46 year-old man with 3 hours of chest pain. What treatment?

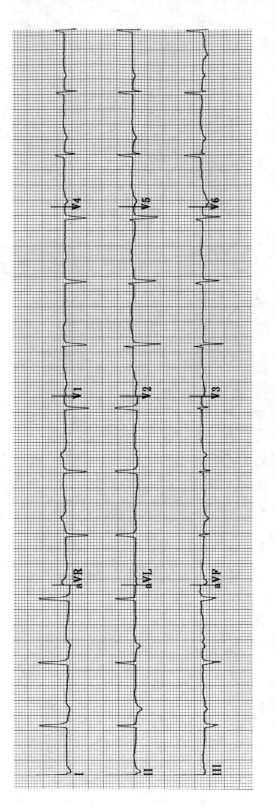

Practice ECG 82   60 year-old woman in good health; routine exam.

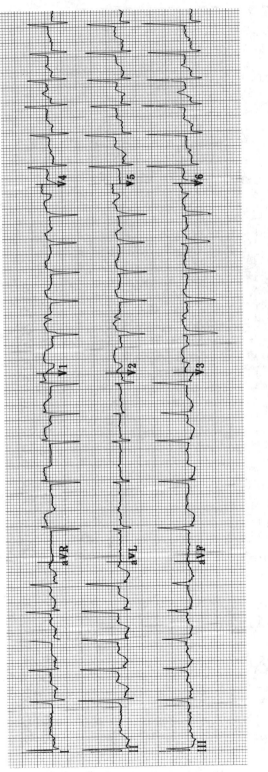

Practice ECG 83 75 year-old woman transferred from a nursing home with dyspnea and pleurisy.

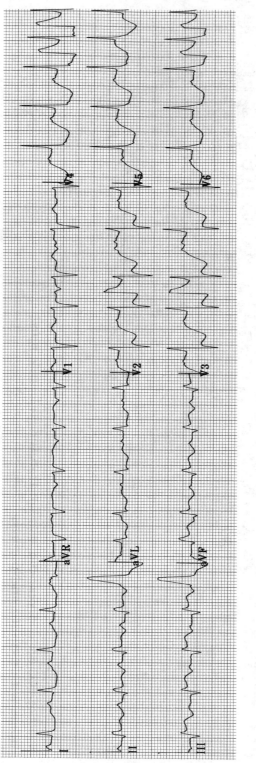

Practice ECG 84 74 year-old man in the emergency room with chest pain that began 30 minutes ago. Is this angina or MI? Is the ischemia anterior or inferior?

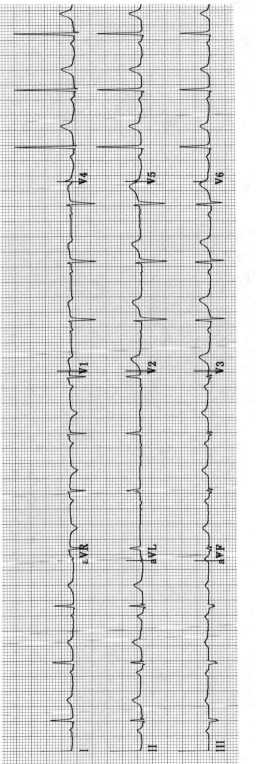

**Practice ECG 85   56 year-old man with no cardiac history; he
wants to start a jogging program.**

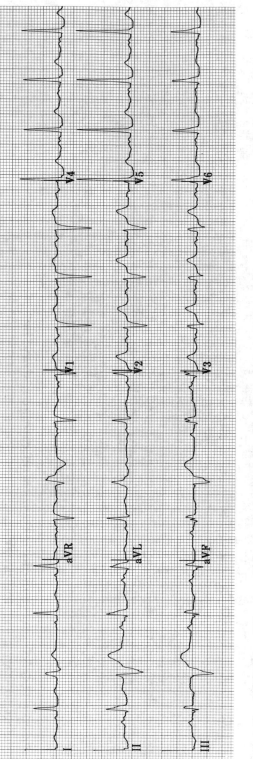

Practice ECG 86   57 year-old man treated for hypertension. Is there evidence of hypertensive heart disease?

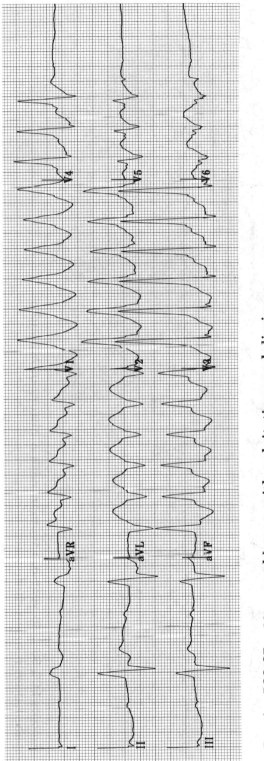

Practice ECG 87   82 year-old man with palpitations and dizziness.

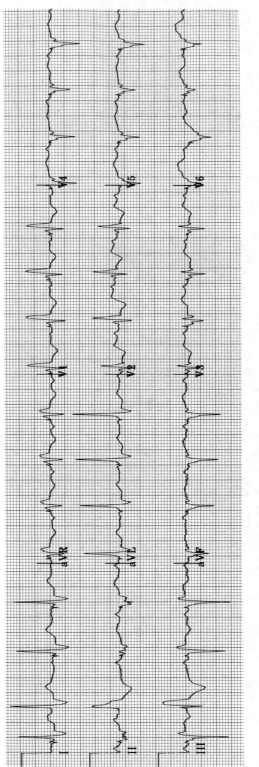
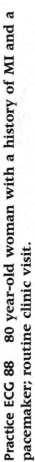

Practice ECG 88 **80 year-old woman with a history of MI and a pacemaker; routine clinic visit.**

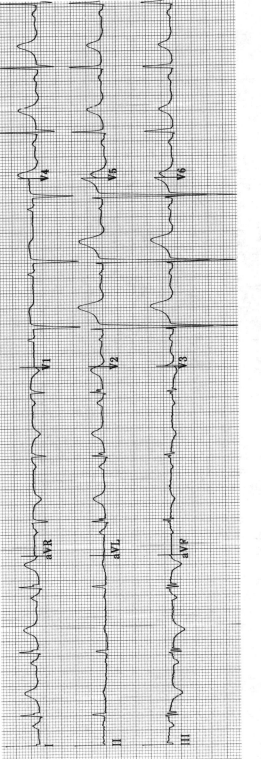

Practice ECG 89   59 year-old woman with intermittent indigestion for 2 weeks.

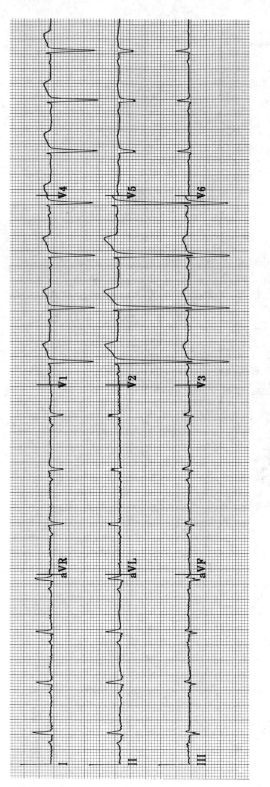

**Practice ECG 90   48 year-old man with a history of inferior MI.
Has he had a second MI?**

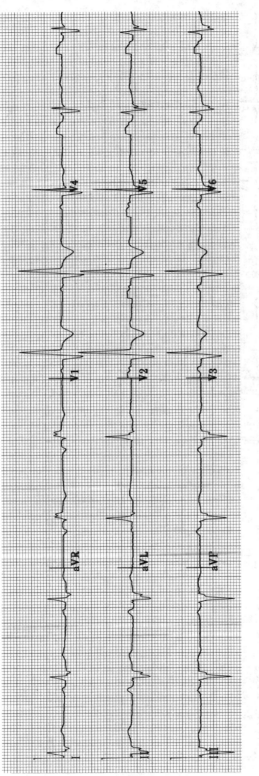
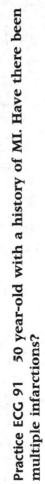

Practice ECG 91   50 year-old with a history of MI. Have there been multiple infarctions?

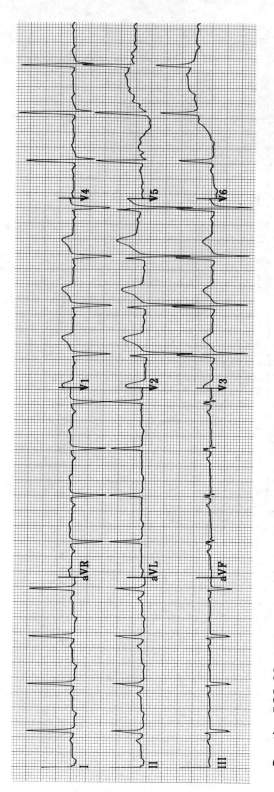

Practice ECG 92   56 year-old man; preoperative ECG.

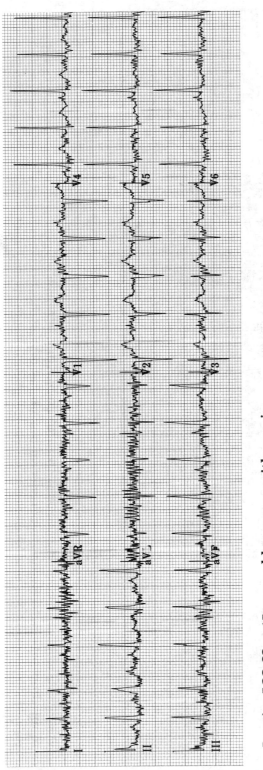

Practice ECG 93   65 year-old woman with sepsis.

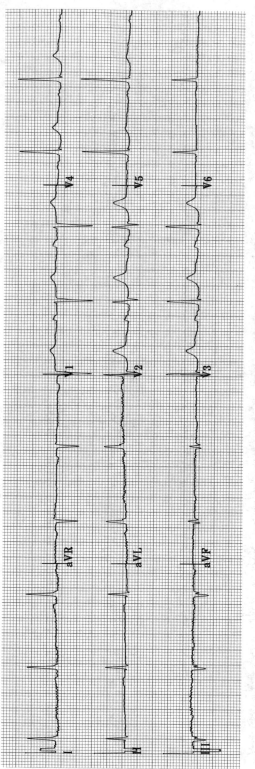

Practice ECG 94   52 year-old man sent to cardiology clinic because of an abnormal ECG. He has hypertension but no history of chest pain.

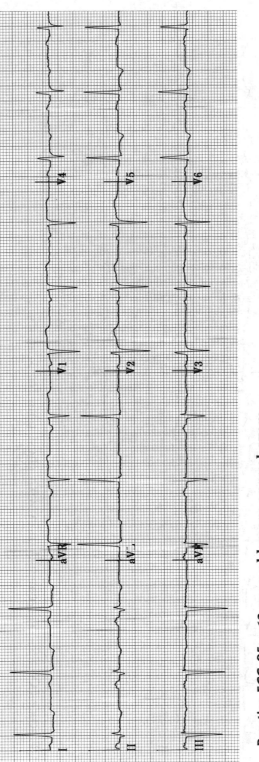

Practice ECG 95   63 year-old man; annual exam.

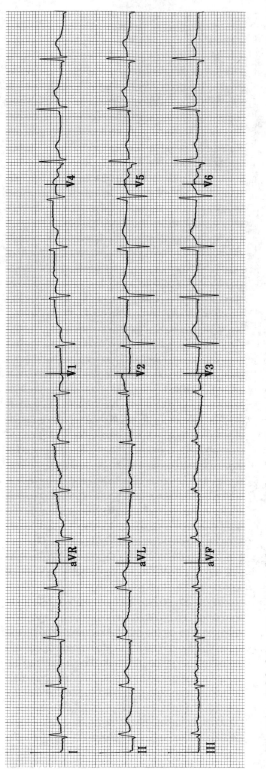

Practice ECG 96 71 year-old man with chest pain for 3 hours.

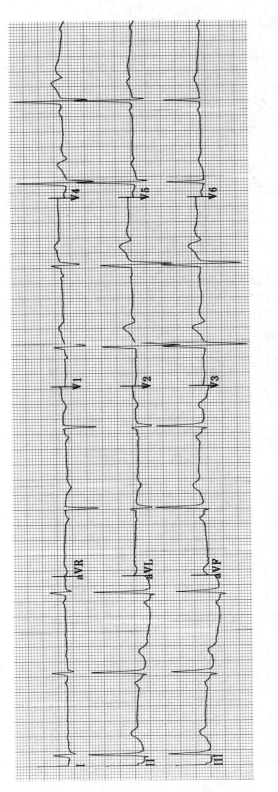

Practice ECG 97   58 year-old man; no clinical data provided.

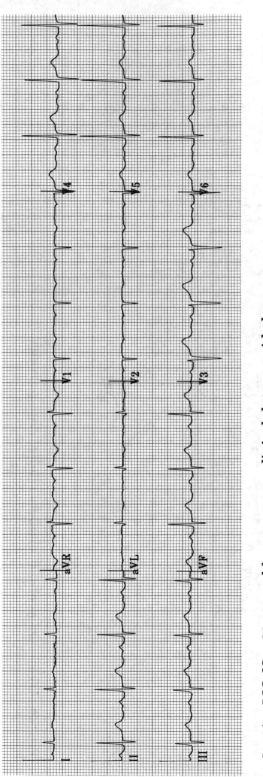

Practice ECG 98   81 year-old woman; no clinical data provided.

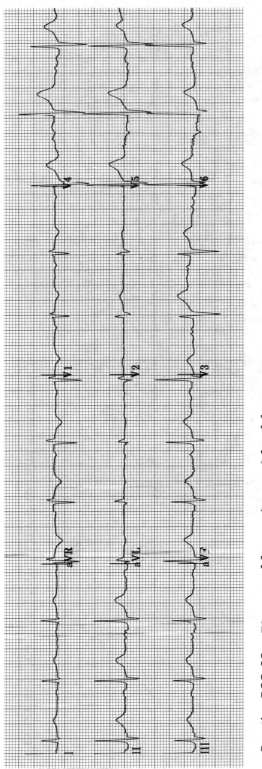

Practice ECG 99   73 year-old man in good health.

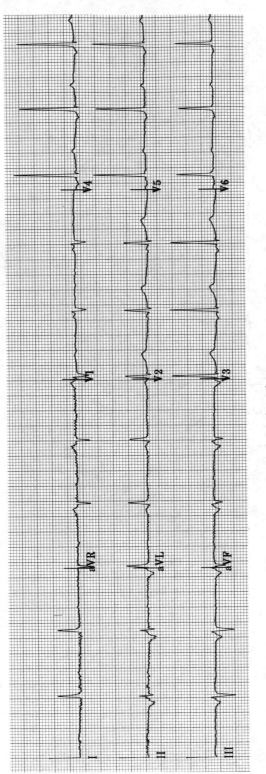

Practice ECG 100   63 year-old man; routine examination.

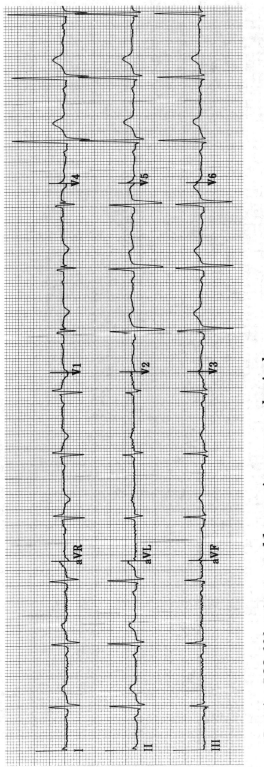

Practice ECG 101   46 year-old man; insurance physical.

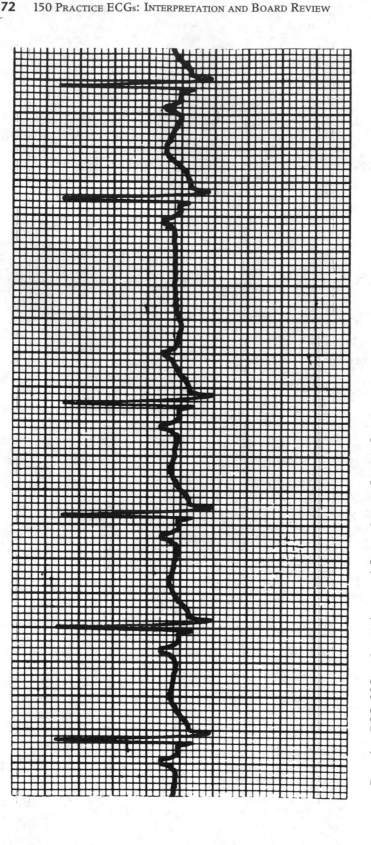

Practice ECG 102   A patient with an irregular pulse.

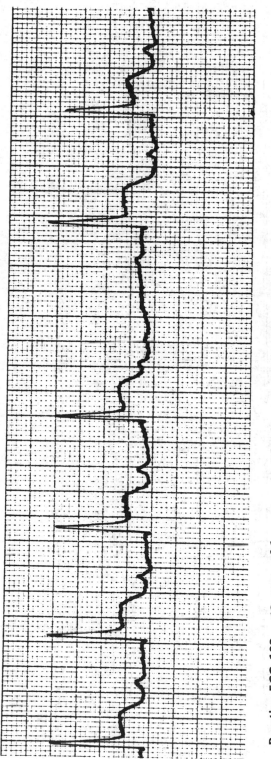

Practice ECG 103   68 year-old woman with acute inferior MI. Does she need a temporary pacemaker?

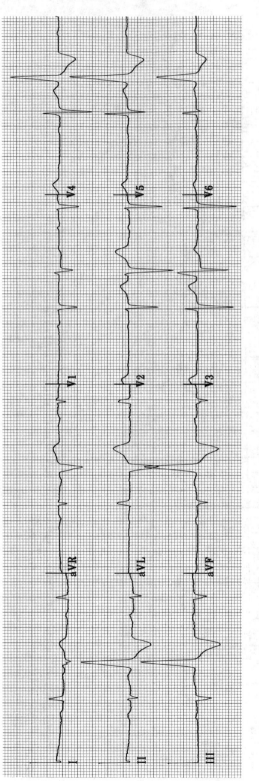

Practice ECG 104   55 year-old man with palpitations and a history of MI.

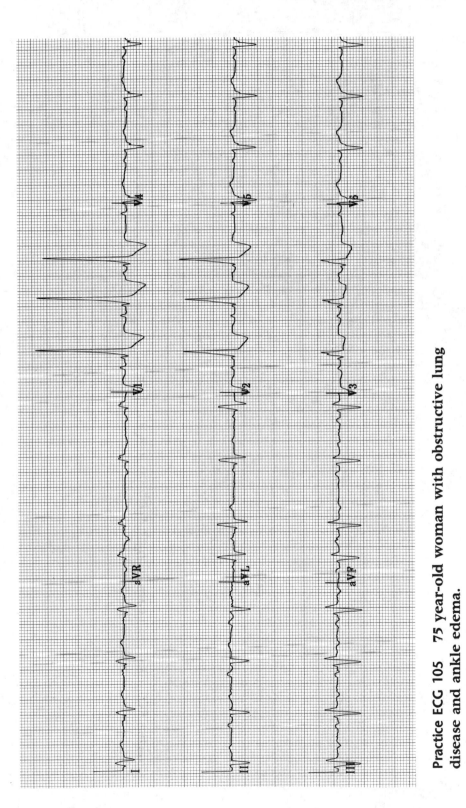

Practice ECG 105   75 year-old woman with obstructive lung disease and ankle edema.

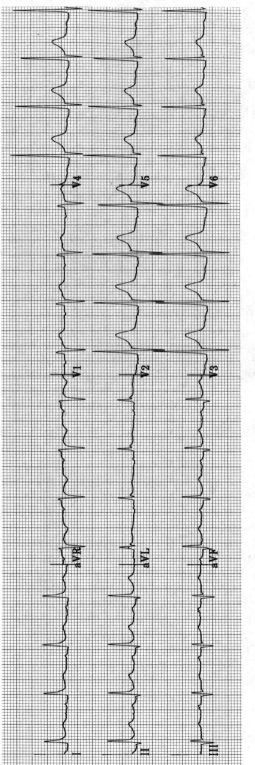

Practice ECG 106   54 year-old man with no history of heart disease. He weighs 275 pounds.

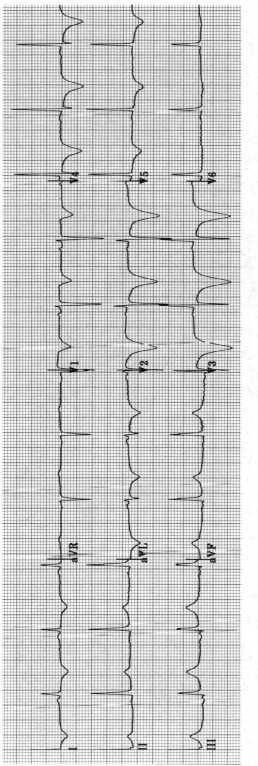

Practice ECG 107 53 year-old man had 90 minutes of chest pain earlier in the day. Should we consider thrombolytic therapy?

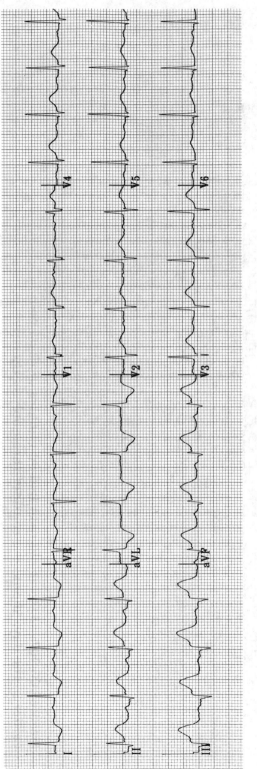

Practice ECG 108   70 year-old woman with chest pain for 5 hours. Should she have thrombolytic therapy?

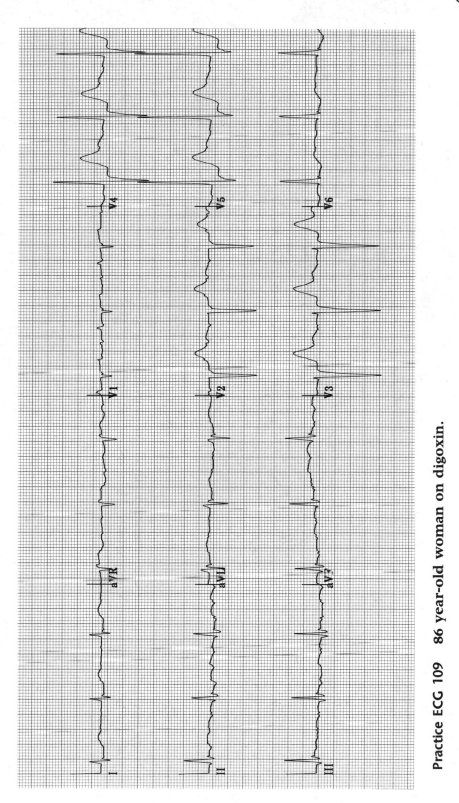

Practice ECG 109   86 year-old woman on digoxin.

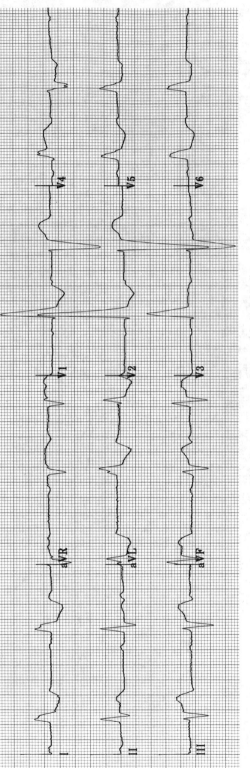

Practice ECG 110   70 year-old woman with chest pain for 2 hours. There is no old ECG for comparison. Should she have thrombolytic therapy?

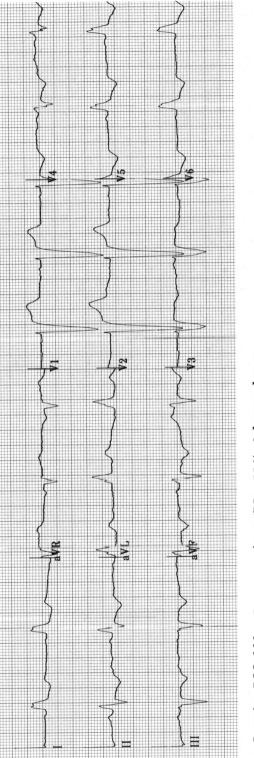

Practice ECG 111   Same patient (No. 110), 3 hours later.

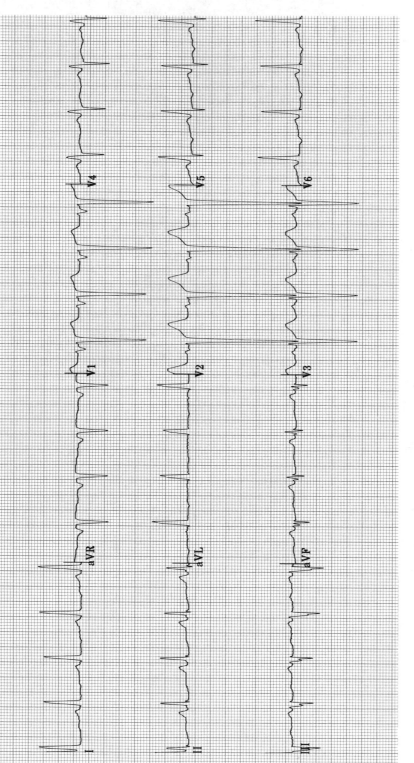

Practice ECG 112   46 year-old man with poorly controlled hypertension and renal failure.

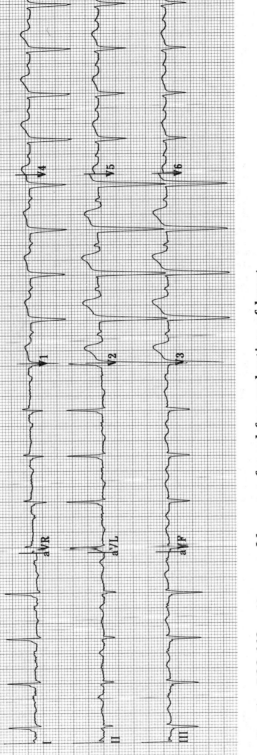
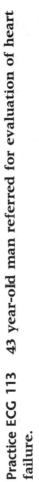

Practice ECG 113 43 year-old man referred for evaluation of heart failure.

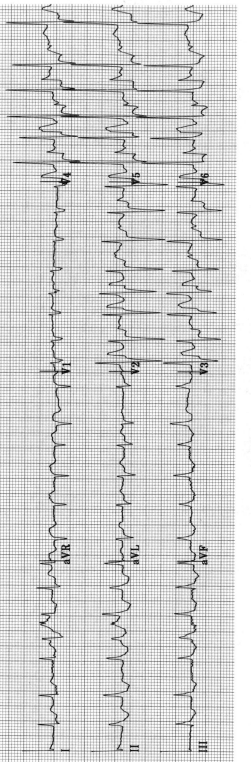
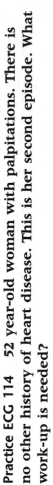

Practice ECG 114   52 year-old woman with palpitations. There is no other history of heart disease. This is her second episode. What work-up is needed?

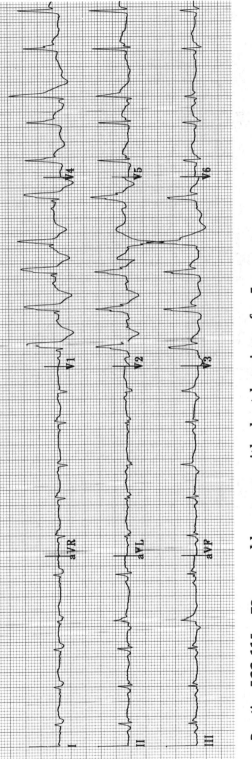

Practice ECG 115   78 year-old woman with chest heaviness for 5 hours and dyspnea. Would thrombolytic therapy influence survival?

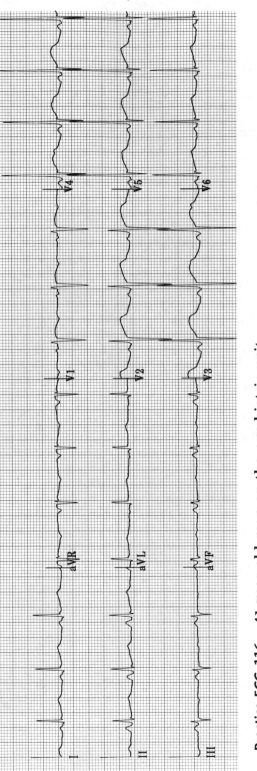

Practice ECG 116   41 year-old man on the psychiatric unit.

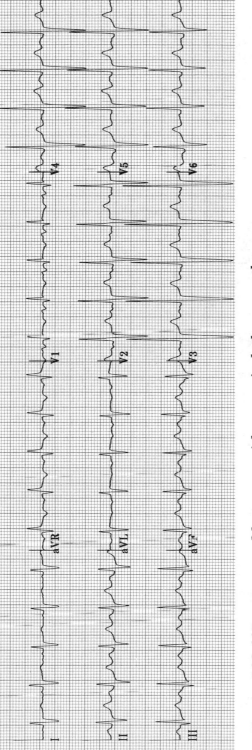

Practice ECG 117 19 year-old woman with cyanosis, lethargy, and a history of heart murmur. What other physical findings would you expect?

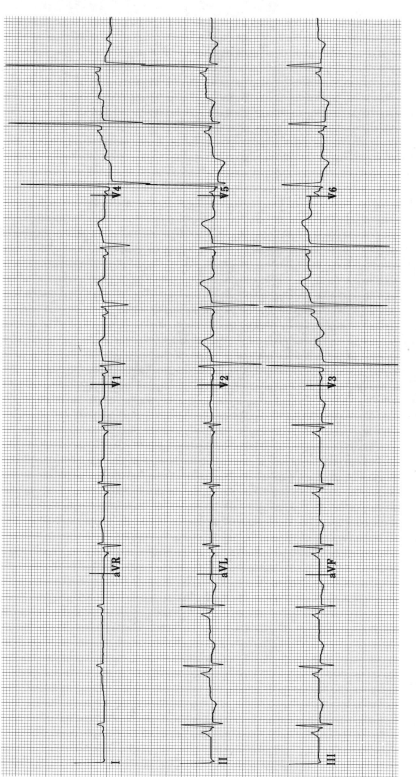

Practice ECG 118   73 year-old man with a systolic murmur that radiates to his neck.

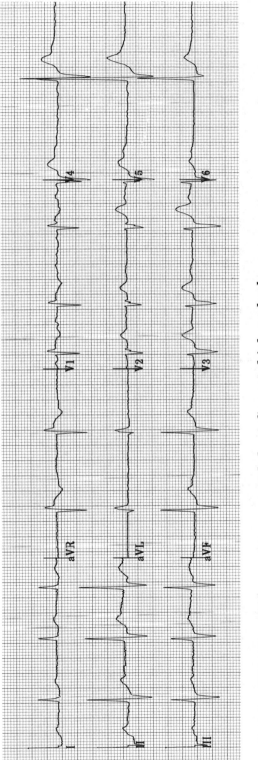

Practice ECG 119 28 year-old man with long fingers, high arched palate, and a diastolic murmur.

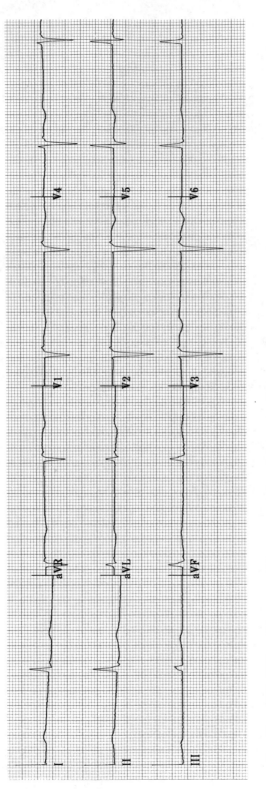

Practice ECG 120 51 year-old man with a history of MI.

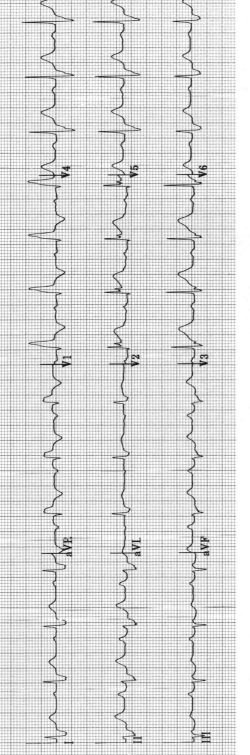

Practice ECG 121 68 year-old man roused from sleep by chest pain 6 hours earlier; antacids did not help. Although the pain is severe, is it too late for reperfusion therapy?

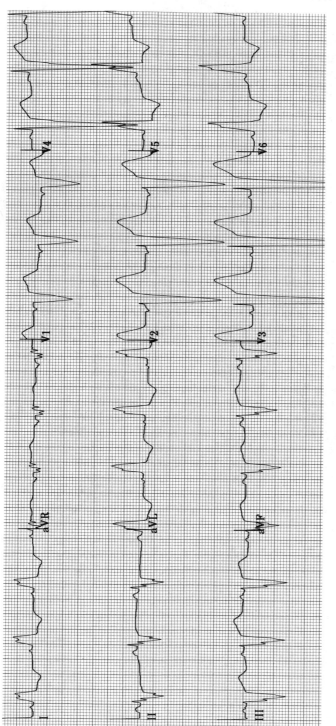

Practice ECG 122   67 year-old woman with a history of hypertension. Is there hypertensive heart disease?

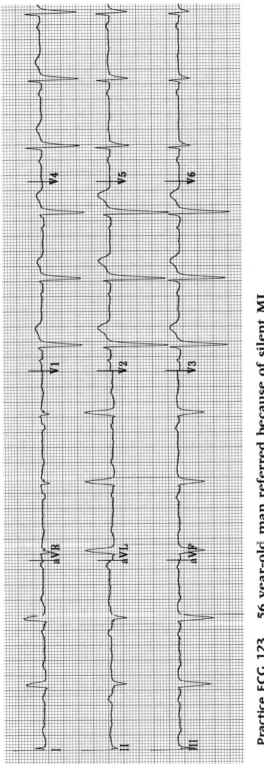
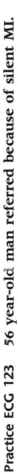

Practice ECG 123   56 year-old man referred because of silent MI.

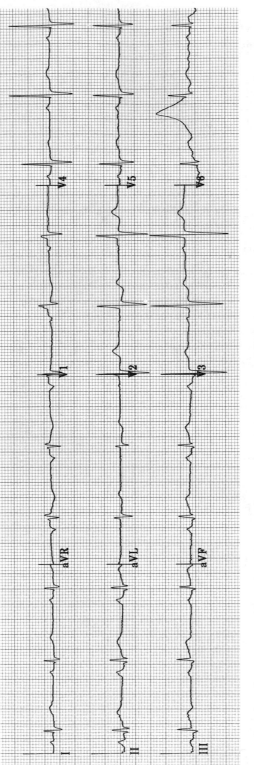

Practice ECG 124   82 year-old woman in good health until the onset of chest pain 2 hours earlier. Should she have thrombolytic therapy?

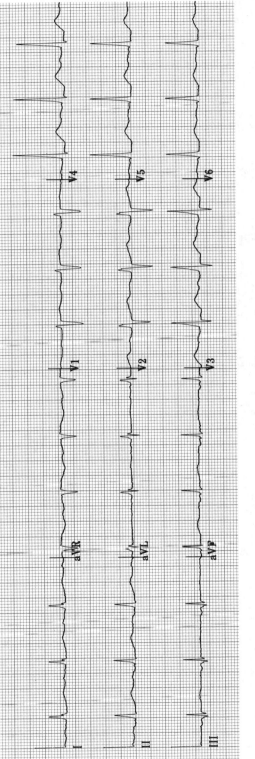

Practice ECG 125   51 year-old woman with hypertension and paroxysmal atrial fibrillation. What medicines is she taking?

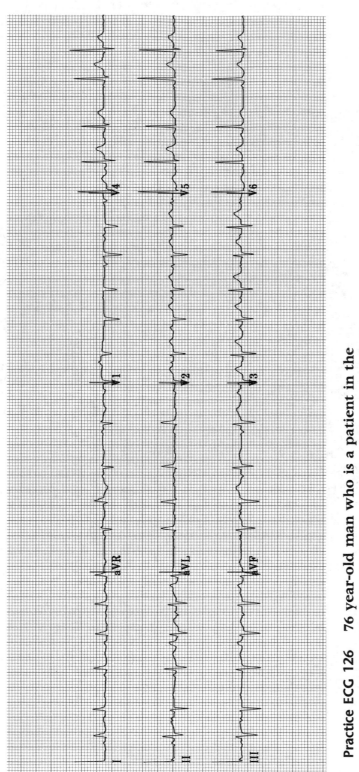

Practice ECG 126 **76 year-old man who is a patient in the pulmonary unit. What medicines could be used to control the heart rate?**

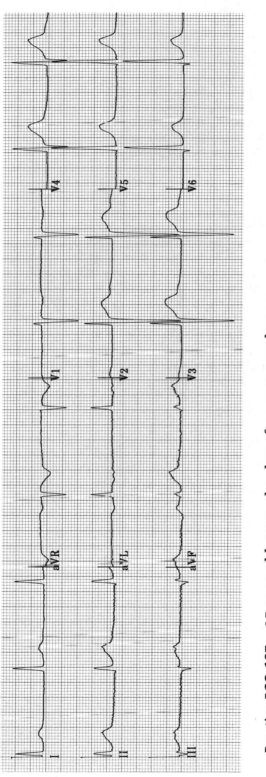

Practice ECG 127   35 year-old man, the day after coronary bypass surgery.

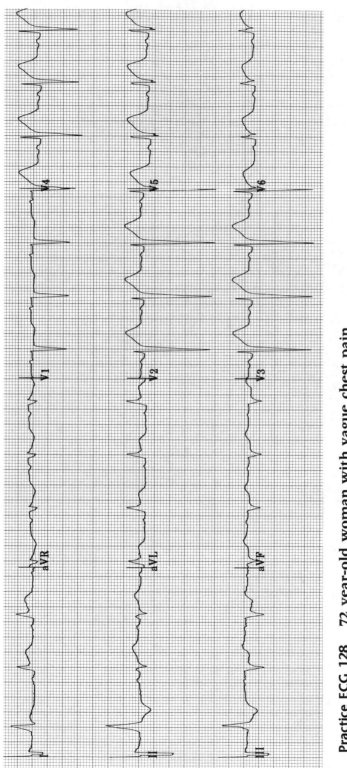

Practice ECG 128   72 year-old woman with vague chest pain unresponsive to antacids.

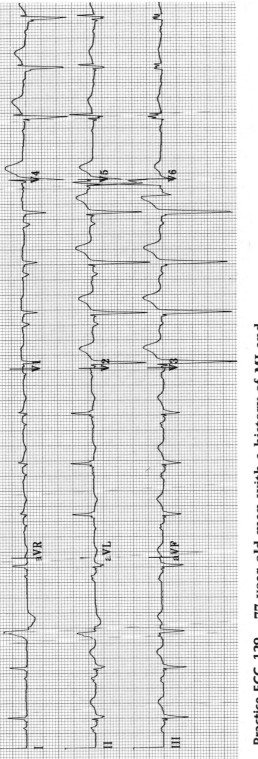

Practice ECG 129　77 year-old man with a history of MI and congestive heart failure.

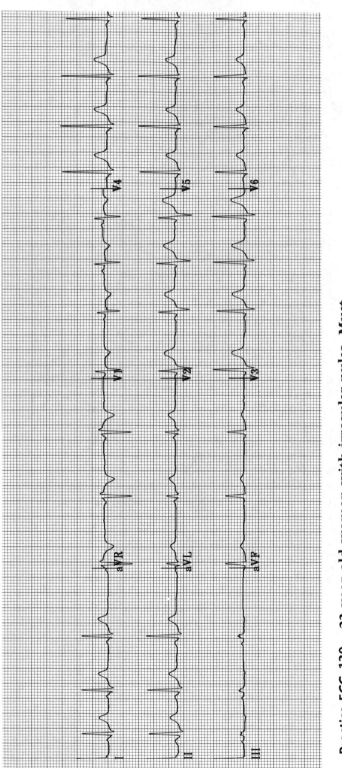

Practice ECG 130   23 year-old woman with irregular pulse. Must we be concerned by this arrhythmia?

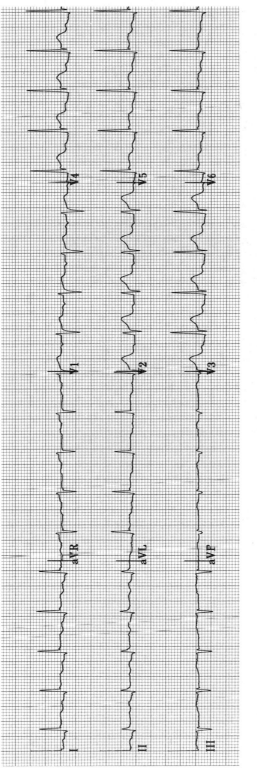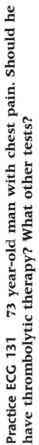

Practice ECG 131   73 year-old man with chest pain. Should he have thrombolytic therapy? What other tests?

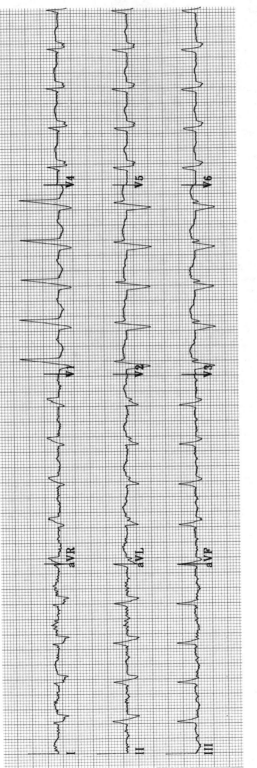
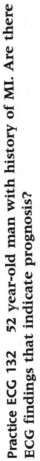

Practice ECG 132   52 year-old man with history of MI. Are there ECG findings that indicate prognosis?

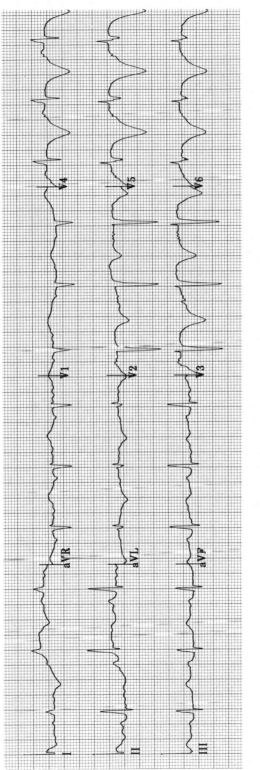

Practice ECG 133   55 year-old woman with confusion, lethargy, and difficulty speaking.

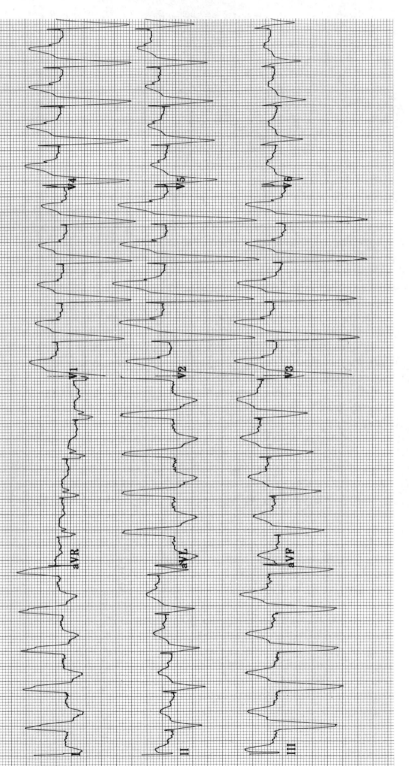

Practice ECG 134   83 year-old woman with heart failure.

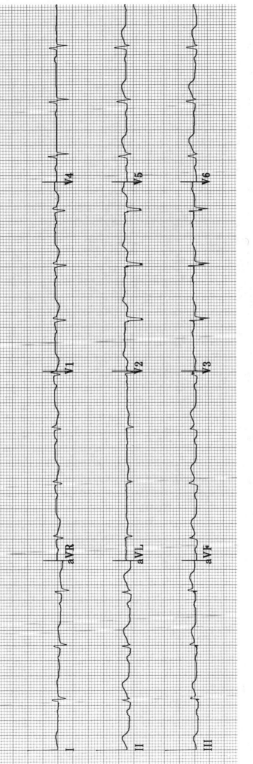

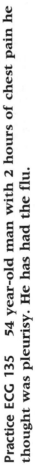

Practice ECG 135 54 year-old man with 2 hours of chest pain he thought was pleurisy. He has had the flu.

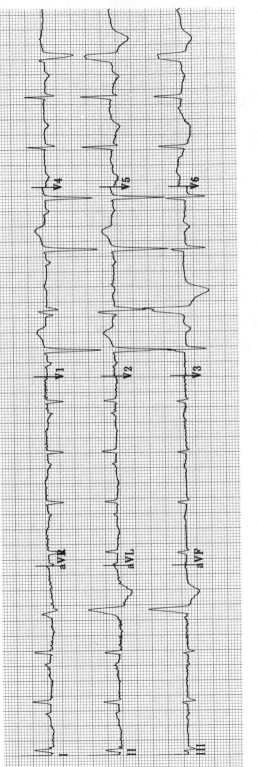
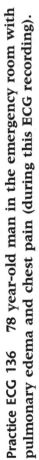

Practice ECG 136   78 year-old man in the emergency room with pulmonary edema and chest pain (during this ECG recording).

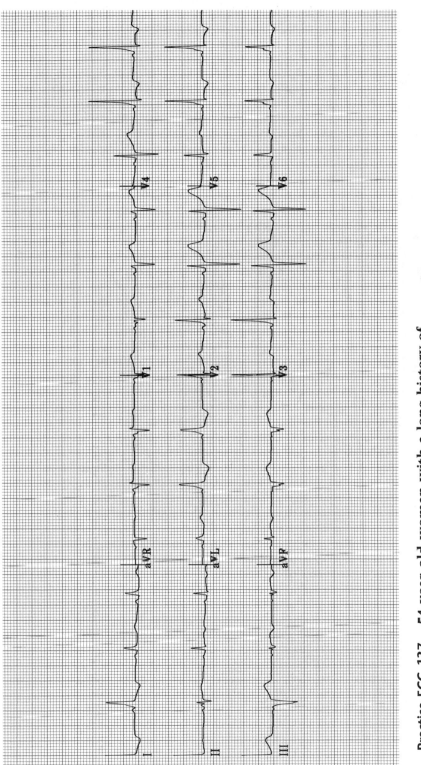

Practice ECG 137   **54 year-old woman with a long history of palpitations; yearly examination.**

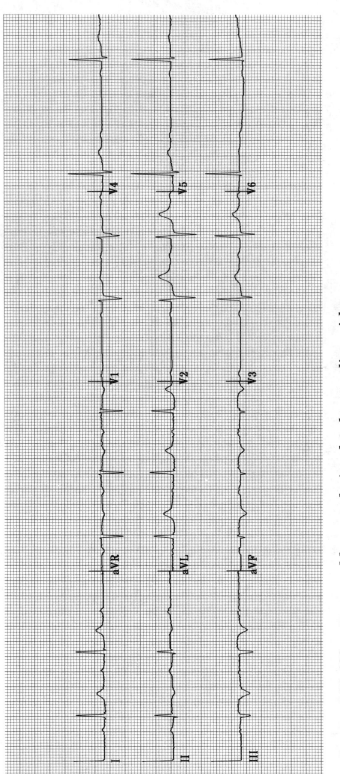
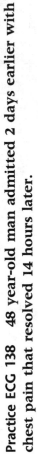

Practice ECG 138 48 year-old man admitted 2 days earlier with chest pain that resolved 14 hours later.

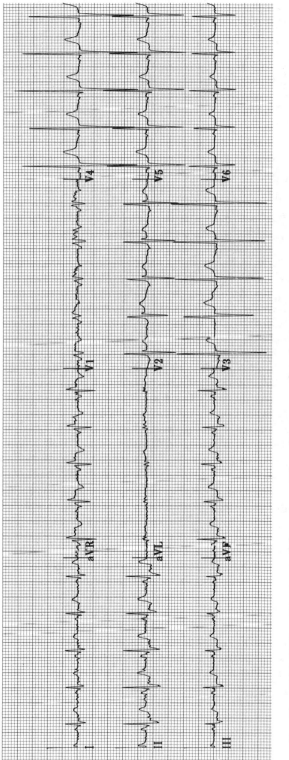

Practice ECG 139   66 year-old man with a history of palpitations. He was admitted with pneumonia and fever.

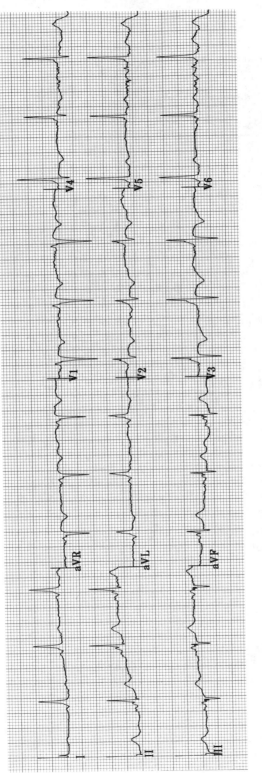

Practice ECG 140   Same patient (No. 139); the pneumonia is being treated and he is afebrile.

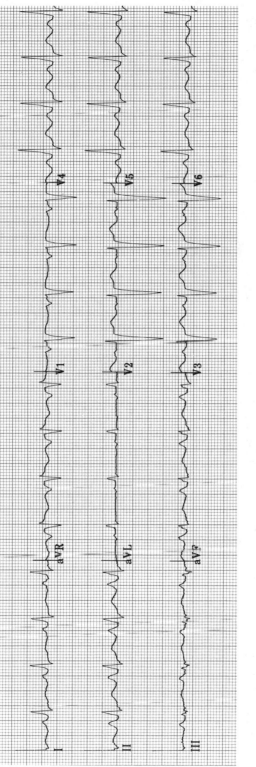

Practice ECG 141　53 year-old woman with a history of hypertension and smoking.

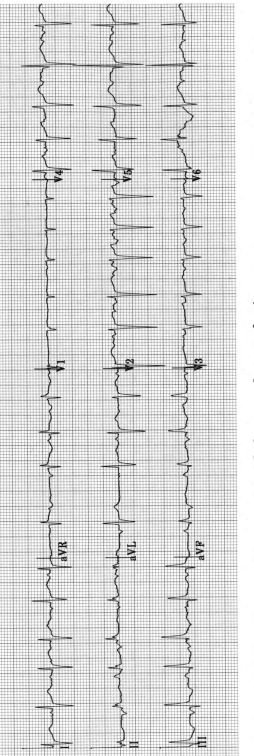
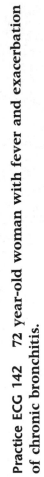

Practice ECG 142   72 year-old woman with fever and exacerbation of chronic bronchitis.

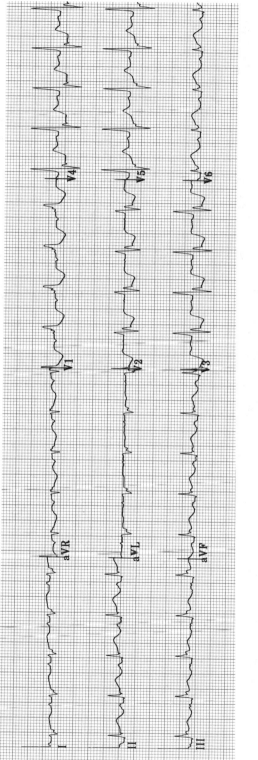

Practice ECG 143   72 year-old man with chest pain for 6 hours. Is there anterior ischemia?

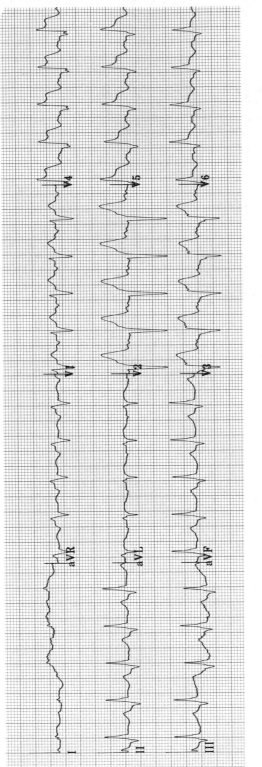

Practice ECG 144   59 year-old man in the emergency room with rales, chest pain, and a systolic blood pressure of 80 mm Hg. What is the correct treatment?

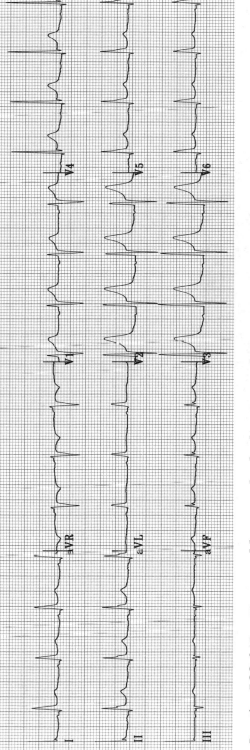

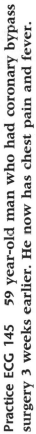

Practice ECG 145 59 year-old man who had coronary bypass surgery 3 weeks earlier. He now has chest pain and fever.

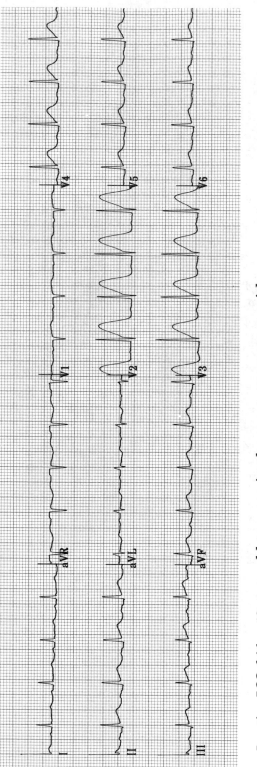
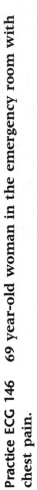

Practice ECG 146   69 year-old woman in the emergency room with chest pain.

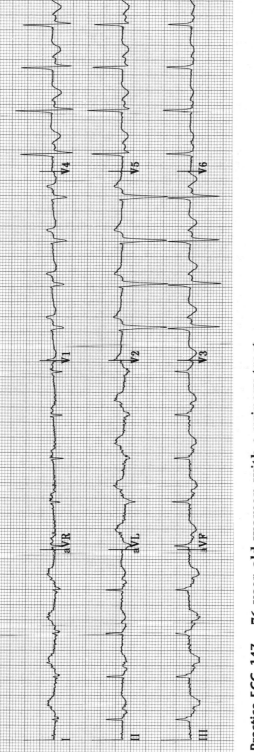

Practice ECG 147   76 year-old woman with a urinary tract infection and possible sepsis.

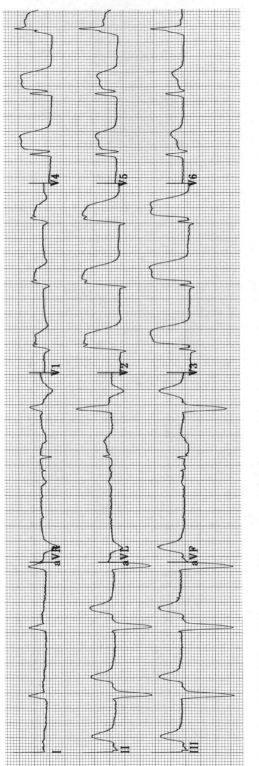

Practice ECG 148   70 year-old man with chest pain.

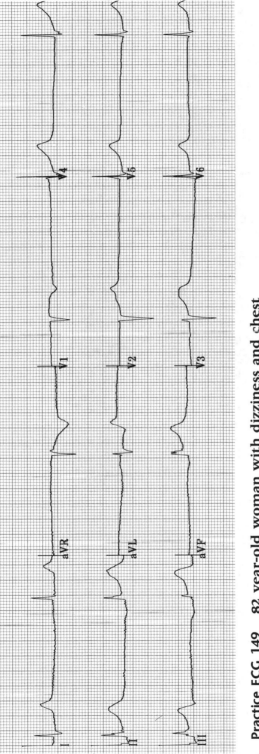

Practice ECG 149   82 year-old woman with dizziness and chest pain.

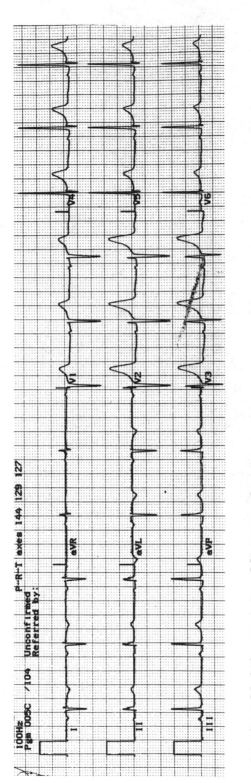

Practice ECG 150   24 year-old ECG technician.

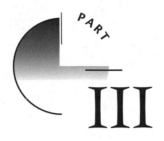

PART

III

Practice ECGs:

Interpretation

and

Comments

The interpretation (I) is the report that accompanies the ECG in the medical record. Comments (C) are provided for teaching purposes. With the initial tracings, I will discuss measurements as well as diagnosis. This will be less necessary with later ECGs.

1. I: Normal sinus rhythm (NSR) 70/min. PR .16, QRS .06, QT normal for the rate. Axis 30°. Normal ECG.

C: There is a P before each QRS, so the rhythm is sinus. Rate—there are just over 4 large squares between R waves (the RR interval); the rate calculation is 300/4 = 75, and because the RR is just above 4 large squares, the rate is a bit lower, about 70/min. QT interval—it is less than half the RR interval, roughly normal. Axis—refer to Fig 1.2. The QRS is almost isoelectric in III (positive and negative forces canceling each other), so the QRS vector is about 90° from lead III, or +30°. Actually, the negative Q wave in III is slightly bigger than the R wave, so the axis may be closer to 25°. Morphology—there is baseline artifact in V₆ that is not worth mentioning. An isolated Q wave in III is a normal finding; inferior MI requires Q's in multiple inferior leads. Note the 1.0-mV standardization deflection at the far left of the tracing; this may be excluded from subsequent tracings. A normal ECG! When you read ECG's in the hospital, you may be surprised to find that normal tracings are outnumbered by those with pathology.

2. I: NSR 60/min. PR .16, QRS .10, QT normal for rate. Axis −35°. Abnormal due to left axis deviation (LAD), intraventricular conduction delay (IVCD), nonspecific T wave changes (NSST-TCs).

C: Rate—the RR interval is 5 large squares (300/5 = 60). Axis—the QRS is roughly isoelectric, a little negative, in II; 90° from II is either −30° or +150°. Because the vector is positive in (points at) I and aVL, the axis is about −30°. I am calling it −35° because the QRS is slightly negative in II. Morphology—because the QRS duration is 0.10 sec and there is slight notching of the QRS in V₁ and V₂, I indicated an IVCD. The QRS is not wide enough for bundle branch block (BBB). T's are inverted in V₅ and V₆, and flat in the inferior (II, III, aVF) and lateral (I and aVL) leads. The cause of the T wave changes is uncertain. In this ECG, the transition from net negative to positive complexes occurs around V₄ and V₅; it is borderline and I elected not to call PRWP.

3. I: Sinus tachycardia (ST), 105/min. PR .14, QRS .08, QT normal for the rate. Axis 0°. Abnormal due to ST and NSST-TCs.

C: Rate—the RR is just under 3 large squares (300/3 = 100). Axis—the QRS is roughly isoelectric in aVF; 90° from aVF is 0°, and the QRS is positive in I. Morphology—the T waves are flat in lateral leads, and there is minimal ST depression.

4. I: NSR, 80/min. PR .12, QRS .08, QT normal for the rate. Axis 90°. Abnormal due to inferior MI of uncertain age.

C: Rate—the RR interval is a bit less than 4 squares (300/4 = 75). Axis—the QRS is isoelectric in I (so the axis is 90° from I), and it is positive in aVF. This is within the normal range, but an axis between 90° and 110° may be called a *vertical* axis. Morphology—there are deep Q waves in II, III, and aVF, strongly suggesting an inferior wall scar. There are other conditions that may cause Q waves, but they are rare (e.g., pre-excitation and hypertrophic cardiomyopathy). Without ST elevation and chest pain, this is not a pattern of acute MI (with ongoing ischemia). It could be a tracing obtained a day (or a month or year) after a completed infarction or successful thrombolytic therapy.

5. I: ST 120/min. PR .16, QRS .08, QT normal for rate. Axis 70°. Abnormal due to the rhythm, anterior infarction and ST depression consistent with ischemia. Since the prior tracing, the ST depression is new.

C: Axis—it is closest to isoelectric, but a bit negative in aVL, which would push the axis to the right of 60°. Morphology—Q's limited to V_1 and V_2 may be called a *septal* MI, but *anterior* is fine. Based on coronary anatomy, it is impossible to have infarction of just the interventricular septum, because septal branches originate from the left anterior descending artery, which also supplies the anterior wall. Nevertheless, the term *septal MI* has traditionally been applied to Q waves limited to V_1 and V_2. The deeply depressed, downsloping ST's in the anterior and lateral leads are more than nonspecific changes: they look ischemic (see Fig 2.10). Furthermore, comparison with a prior ECG (not provided here) showed that the ST changes were new, and the patient was having chest pain. In this clinical context, the diagnosis of active ischemia is almost certain, but it is a diagnosis that should be made by the clinician, not the ECG reader. This interpretation goes far enough, although I suggest clinical correlation could be added.

6. I: NSR 80/min. PR .12, QRS .09, QT normal. Axis 80°. Probably normal ECG with small inferior Q's noted, and diffuse J-point elevation (consider early repolarization).

C: Axis—there is no lead with an isoelectric QRS. To be negative in aVL, the axis has to be more than 60°, and to be positive in I, less than 90°. So the axis is between 60° and 90°, but closer to 90° as it is so negative in aVL. For a Q wave to be significant, it should be a box deep and a box wide. These inferior Q's do not make it; I mention them to make it clear they were not overlooked.

The *J point* is the junction between the QRS and the ST segment. In this case, it is above the baseline in V_2 through V_6, and minimally so in inferior and lateral leads. The ST segments are elevated but maintain normal shape with upward concavity. This ST elevation is worth mention, but it should be interpreted in clinical context. For a patient in the emergency room with chest pain, it could indicate pericarditis (it involves multiple vascular distributions, and normal upward concavity is maintained); you could not be sure from this tracing. Because you know that this is an insurance examination and that he is young, early repolarization is a safe guess (and it is identified as a guess on the report).

7. I: Supraventricular tachycardia (SVT) 160/min, PR uncertain, QRS .06, QT nor-

mal. Axis −50°. Abnormal due to SVT, left anterior fascicular block (LAFB), anterior MI of uncertain age, and low voltage.

C: Rhythm—it is a narrow complex tachycardia (with narrow QRS's) and no obvious P waves (could they be buried in the T wave in lead II?). It is a bit too fast for ST in an elderly person; SVT is a reasonable call, and it would include ST as well as other supraventricular tachyarrhythmias. Axis—to be negative in II, it has to be left of −30°, and I am guessing far to the left (beyond −45°), which makes it LAFB. There are deep Q's in V_1 through V_3; most with this finding have had an MI, although false positives are possible.

8. I: NSR 70/min. PR .16, QRS .08, QT normal. Axis 10°. Abnormal due to anterior MI and probably inferior MI of uncertain age and nonspecific T wave changes.

C: Axis—almost isoelectric, but a bit negative in III, so the axis is to the left of 30°; strongly positive in aVF, so it is to the right of 0°. There are Q's in V_1 and V_2. MI is the correct interpretation, although it could be a false positive. The Q in aVF is broad, although not deep, and there is the deep Q in III. T's are flat in I, aVL, and V_5 and V_6. Heart failure may be attributed to ischemic cardiomyopathy in a patient with Q waves in two of the three coronary artery distributions.

9. I: NSR 75/min. PR .22, QRS .11, QT normal. Axis −50°. Abnormal due to first-degree AV block (1°AVB), LAFB, incomplete right bundle branch block (IRBBB), and left ventricular hypertrophy (LVH) with repolarization changes.

C: If you did not measure the PR, you probably missed the 1°AVB, as the P waves are not prominent. Axis—the QRS is deeply negative in II, so the axis is far left of −30°; it is slightly negative in aVR, placing the axis just to the right of −60°. I count 7 points for LVH (see Table 2.1): voltage (deep S in III), prolonged QRS, delayed intrinsicoid deflection (look at aVL, a good example of the delay in the time to reach peak voltage), and LAD. The ST-T changes in V_4 through V_6 are probably due to LVH, but it is not the classic strain pattern. A couple of problems with this ECG: Why not inferior MI? There are small positive glitches, R waves, in inferior leads, so there are no Q's. What about the tall R in V_1? Look closely at that lead: at first glance, the QRS looks narrower than in V_2. V_1 actually has an rsR pattern, not quite RBBB, as the QRS is not wide enough—but close (I call it IRBBB). LAFB + RBBB would not change the final diagnosis of LVH.

Would bifascicular block plus 1°AVB raise the possibility of incipient trifascicular (complete) heart block and syncope? Not necessarily, as most patients with this pattern are found to have PR prolongation because of delayed conduction within the AV node, not below it in the left posterior fascicle. Syncope is a symptom that is more common in elderly patients, but this tracing does not indicate a need for a pacemaker or electrophysiologic study in the absence of symptoms.

10. I: NSR 95/min. PR .24, QRS .08, QT normal. Axis 0°. Abnormal due to 1°AVB.

C: Axis—the QRS is isoelectric in aVF and the vector is aimed at lead I (most strongly positive in I). Where should you measure the PR interval? Where the P is well seen and the interval seems longest (lead V$_3$). Notice that the P is buried in the down-slope of the T wave in II, making the QT appear a bit longer in that lead. None of these findings explains her loss of memory.

11. I: Atrial fibrillation (AF) about 70/min with PVCs or aberrantly conducted supra-ventricular beats. QRS .10, QT normal. Axis −50°. Abnormal due to AF, LAFB, and possible inferior MI.

C: Fibrillation waves are seen in V$_1$ and the rhythm is grossly irregular; the rate is a bit slower than usual with AF (consider a digoxin level). Axis—the QRS is slightly negative in aVR and negative in II, putting the axis between −30° and −60°; it looks closer to −60° to me. Are there inferior Q's? The one in III is definite, but there may be a tiny positive glitch in the first complex in aVF, so I hedged with the diagnosis of inferior MI. We do not see much of the ectopic complexes at the end of the recording. Their initial vectors are similar to the other QRS complexes; they could be aberrantly conducted supraventricular beats.

12. I: AF 80/min. QRS .10, QT normal, Axis 45°. Abnormal due to AF, high QRS voltage, and nonspecific ST-T changes (probably digitalis effect). Cannot exclude LVH.

C: Axis—the QRS is positive in all limb leads except aVR; with it positive in aVL and III, the axis must be between 30° and 60°. When all the limb leads are positive, save aVR, I call it 45°. The deep S in V$_2$ meets voltage criteria for LVH, but the ST changes count less because of digoxin therapy. There may be LVH, and there prob-ably is with the history of hypertension and presence of AF, but a definite diagnosis cannot be made from this ECG. These ST segment changes are typical of digitalis effect; they sag as if you hooked them with your finger and dragged them down. This is different from the ST depression of ischemia (see ECG No. 5) or LV strain (see Fig 2.5). It is a safe bet this patient is taking digoxin (AF and a controlled ventricular rate plus these ST changes).

13. I: NSR 80/min, PR .18, QRS .08, QT normal. Axis 20°. Borderline ECG with NSST-TCs noted.

C: Axis—QRS slightly negative in III, the axis is just to the left of 30°. The flat T's and sagging ST's in V$_3$ through V$_5$ are not quite normal.

14. I: NSR 90/min. PR .18, QRS .16, QT prolonged for the rate (QTc .53). Axis −30°. Abnormal due to left atrial abnormality (LAA), LAD, RBBB, LVH with repolarization abnormalities, and QT interval prolongation.

C: Axis—the QRS is isoelectric in II. LAA—there is a terminal, negative deflection in the P in V$_1$ plus notching of the P in inferior leads. LVH—voltage, LAA, LAD, wide QRS, and ST-T changes. The QT interval is definitely longer than half the RR interval.

15. I: NSR 60/min. PR .16, QRS .10, QT normal. Axis 35°. Abnormal due to anterior MI of uncertain age and NSST-TCs.

C: Axis—the QRS is roughly isoelectric in III, perhaps a shade positive. There are deep Q's in V_1 through V_3, with associated T inversion. Because the T inversion extends to lateral leads (V_5 and V_6, I, and aVL), I added NSST-TCs to the interpretation, but these changes are probably a part of the MI pattern. Thrombolytic therapy? No, because there is no ST elevation, the usual marker of acute, transmural ischemia. You need old tracings for comparison, and you should consider other causes of chest pain. In general, when a patient has recurrent ischemic symptoms, they are identical to those from previous events. I always ask, "Is this just like the pain you had during your heart attack?" If this patient's pain is ischemic, this ECG suggests that it is angina rather than acute MI—try nitroglycerine therapy. But antacids may work!

16. I: Atrial fibrillation, about 90/min. QRS .11, QT normal. Axis −10°. Abnormal due to AF, IVCD, and LVH with associated ST-T changes.

C: Axis—almost isoelectric, but a bit negative in aVF. QT interval—the Bazett calculation falls apart with a variable RR interval. In complexes with long RR intervals (V_6 or III), the QT is well below half the RR. When the RR is short, the QT seems long. It is a problem with AF; to diagnose long QT, I want the QT to seem long regardless of the RR. LVH—voltage in V_2, ST-T changes, wide QRS, and delayed intrinsicoid deflection.

Should she be treated for isolated systolic hypertension? Yes—the Systolic Hypertension in the Elderly Program found that the degree of systolic pressure elevation correlated best with development of LVH, heart failure, stroke, and death; diastolic pressure was less important. Based on the ECG, this patient already has hypertensive heart disease. An echocardiogram probably would confirm increased LV thickness.

17. I: NSR 75/min. PR .18, QRS .08, QT normal. Axis −30°. Borderline due to left axis deviation.

C: Axis—the QRS is isoelectric in II. It is a fair interpretation; the axis is on the left border of the normal range, but that is the only abnormality. Do not take the *abnormal* designation lightly, particularly for a young patient. An abnormal ECG may mean *heart disease* to his insurance company or employer.

18. NSR 60/min. PR .20, QRS .10, QT-U prolonged for the rate. Axis −15°. Abnormal due to poor R wave progression (PRWP), possible inferior MI, U wave and QT-U prolongation, and possible LVH with associated ST-T changes.

C: Axis—the QRS is positive in II and negative in aVF, which places the axis between 0° and −30°. U wave—well seen in V_3 through V_6. LVH—wide QRS and ST-T changes in I and aVL. Voltage is close to meeting LVH criteria in the limb leads. The ST-T changes may be missing in V_5 and V_6 because of PRWP—a dilated heart is one of the causes of PRWP, and LV changes may be displaced to the left of V_6, just as the apical impulse may be displaced to the left (perhaps there would be T wave inversion if there were a lead V_8). You notice, however, that I hedge on the diagnosis of LVH. A conduction abnormality, common in elderly patients, could be responsible for T wave changes, delayed transition, and the wide QRS. In this case, make the diagnosis of LVH with an echocardiogram, not the ECG. There is nothing on this ECG that explains her dizziness. There are Q waves in two of the three inferior leads.

19. I: NSR 70/min. PR .16, QRS .10, QT normal. Axis 70°. Abnormal ECG due to possible inferior MI and NSST-TCs. Clinical correlation needed.

C: Axis—the QRS is almost isoelectric, but a bit negative, in aVL. The Q waves in inferior leads are small, on the borderline for the diagnosis of MI. The T's are a bit tall and peaked in anterior leads, and the T axis is opposite the QRS axis in those leads, but this probably is a normal finding. There is J-point elevation in the V leads. Asking for clinical correlation could apply to every ECG you read, but for tracings with borderline findings, it is worth mention on the report (it is more than just another way to hedge).

20. I: NSR 70/min. PR .24, QRS .09, QT normal. Axis −30°. Abnormal due to 1°AVB, LAD, and inferolateral MI of uncertain age.

C: When compared to the previous case, this patient's Q waves are deeper and wider and are found in all three of the inferior leads. The diagnosis of inferior MI is certain. There are also deep Q's in V_5 and V_6, lateral leads. Perhaps he has had two MI's with occlusion of the artery to the inferior wall, then occlusion of another vessel to the lateral wall. But this is unlikely. Instead, the coronary artery supplying this patient's inferior wall probably was large, wrapping around the heart and supplying a part of the lateral wall as well. The resulting infarct was large enough to leave him with heart failure. Inferior MI is usually smaller and less consequential than anterior infarction; this case may be an exception.

21. I: NSR 80/min. PR .13, QRS .09, QT normal. Axis 100°. Abnormal due to biatrial abnormality, PRWP, and right ventricular hypertrophy.

C: RAA is obvious (tall P's in inferior leads); LAA is arguable, as there is no positive deflection before the negative deflection in V_1. RVH—tall R in V_1, deep S in V_6, T inversion in V_1 (the strain pattern), RAD, right atrial abnormality (RAA). Based on physical findings and the ECG, the patient probably has tricuspid regurgitation.

22. I: ST 130/min. PR .14, QRS .08, QTc .40. Axis 90°. Abnormal due to ST, right atrial abnormality, PRWP, and NSST-TCs. Small inferior Q's noted.

C: The tall, peaked P waves are typical. She does not meet criteria for RVH. But the axis, RAA, PRWP, and relatively low voltage make emphysema a good possibility. Sinus tachycardia suggests that the patient is struggling; within hours of this ECG, she was on a ventilator.

23. I: Atrial flutter and a ventricular pacemaker at 70/min.

C: The sawtooth flutter waves are apparent in inferior leads. Look at the QRS complexes in I and II; there is a small pacing spike at the beginning of each. The pacer must be located in the right ventricle, as there is a LBBB pattern. The QRS morphology of the paced beat is not usually mentioned in the formal interpretation.

A demand, ventricular pacemaker is commonly set to pace at about 70/min. It is designated a VVI pacemaker: *v*entricular sensing, *v*entricular pacing, and programmed to be *i*nhibited from pacing if it senses a native QRS.

24. I: NSR 65/min with an isolated PVC. PR .18, QRS .08, QT normal. Axis 45°. Abnormal due to LAA, and probable LVH.

C: The P wave is biphasic in V_1 and is probably notched in inferior leads. Axis—the QRS is positive in all limb leads (save aVR). LVH—criteria include voltage, LAA, and borderline ST changes. Is there an infarct pattern? I think there are small, positive glitches, R waves, before the S waves in II and aVF (may be wrong).

Although there is probable LVH, he does not have the typical strain pattern seen with the pressure overload caused by aortic stenosis. Volume overload causes LV dilatation and an increase in LV mass without a big increase in LV thickness. This man had mitral regurgitation with a dilated but not thickened LV. The ECG does not make the differentiation, but the findings are consistent with the diagnosis.

25. I: Nodal rhythm, 58/min. QRS .13, QT long for the rate. Axis about 10°. Abnormal due to a long QTc, rhythm, and RBBB.

C: Retrograde P's are seen at the beginning of the T wave in multiple leads. The QT seems quite long in V_4 and V_5, and the calculated QTc is .55 sec. Thiazide diuretics may depress potassium and/or magnesium levels, causing prolongation of the QT interval. It is important to diagnose and correct these electrolyte disturbances, as they may lead to ventricular arrhythmias and sudden death. Check a digoxin level as well, as the nodal rhythm may be evidence of digitalis toxicity.

26. I: ST 108/min. PR .16, QRS .08, QT normal. Axis 70°. Abnormal due to ST, anterior MI of uncertain age with persistent ST elevation.

C: Axis—close to isoelectric, though slightly negative, in aVL. He probably had the MI a month earlier and misinterpreted his symptoms. Resting tachycardia a month after anterior infarction is a worrisome finding suggesting LV dysfunction. That is reason enough for an echocardiogram. In addition, persistent ST elevation in infarct zone leads may indicate an LV aneurysm. This unfortunate fellow should have had reperfusion therapy at the time of his acute MI.

27. I: NSR 60/min. PR .18, QRS .08, QT normal. Axis 45°. Abnormal due to deep T inversion in anterior leads consistent with ischemia or non-Q MI.

C: She should be hospitalized and treated with aspirin, heparin, and antianginal drugs. Cardiac enzymes probably will be elevated, which would make the diagnosis of infarction rather than unstable angina. Angiography is indicated and probably would show a tight and ragged-appearing lesion in the anterior descending coronary artery, possibly with thrombus. Although this infarction is a small one, with only minimal injury to the anterior wall, she is at risk for occlusion and transmural MI.

28. I: NSR 70/min. PR .19, QRS .10, QT normal. Axis −15°. Abnormal due to NSST-TCs; cannot exclude LVH.

C: Axis—the QRS is slightly negative in aVF, positive in II, so the axis is between 0° and −30°. LVH—the QRS is slightly wide and the axis is toward the left, but neither finding achieves significance. Voltage is not high. There is just the lateral T inversion. She may have LVH, and the ECG is just not sensitive enough to make a certain diagnosis. Get an echocardiogram to measure LV thickness.

29. I: AF with rapid ventricular response. QRS .10, QT long for the rate, axis 0°. Abnormal due to AF, LVH with repolarization changes, and inferior MI of uncertain age. Cannot exclude active ischemia.

C: The ST segment depression may all be due to LVH, but the degree of depression seems too deep for that. A rapid ventricular rate can provoke ischemia, which may be painless in a patient with diabetic neuropathy. I would treat her for ischemia as well as pulmonary congestion. (It later became apparent that she had ketoacidosis and pulmonary edema precipitated by a non-Q infarction.)

30. I: NSR 80/min. PR .18, QRS .16, QT normal, axis 100°. Abnormal due to RBBB, RAD, and possibly acute anterior and inferior MI.

C: This is an unusual ECG because there is ST elevation in both inferior and anterior leads. Recall that it is uncommon for acute ischemia to occur simultaneously in two different vascular distributions. Why would two different arteries occlude at the same time? Global ST elevation instead suggests a global etiology such as pericarditis. But this looks more like ischemia to me, because the ST's are upwardly convex, and because there is T inversion at the same time there is ST elevation. The T's can invert with pericarditis, but the ST's usually return to baseline before they do.

Here is the explanation for this case of coincidental MI's. His right coronary artery occluded and he had inferior MI 2 years earlier, but the infarct was incomplete. He had collateral flow from the anterior descending artery to the distal right coronary artery (see Fig 2.8). Although there was injury to the inferior wall, some muscle was saved by the collateral vessels. Now he has occluded the anterior descending artery, losing flow to the anterior wall plus the flow through the collaterals to his inferior wall. He is thus losing two vascular distributions with a single coronary occlusion.

Comparison of this ECG with old tracings showed that the bifascicular block is new; plans were made to take the patient to the catheterization lab for a temporary pacemaker and acute angioplasty. While in the elevator, he lost his blood pressure and died from cardiogenic shock. (Cause of death? How about old age? Multiple infarctions complicated by LV failure is just too much heart disease for an 85 year-

old person. There are many clinicians who would argue against aggressive, inter-
ventional therapy at this stage of life when the odds of success are poor.)

31. I: ST 110/min. PR .14, QRS .16. Axis −20°. Abnormal due to the rhythm and
LBBB.

C: In this case, the QTc is .50 sec. In the presence of LBBB, QT prolongation loses
its significance. There is increased voltage, a wide QRS, and lateral ST-T wave
changes and possibly LAA. However, LBBB also precludes an ECG diagnosis of LVH
(as it does MI). With her history of hypertension and this grossly abnormal ECG,
she probably has hypertensive heart disease and LVH. An echocardiogram would
be needed to make the diagnosis (and has become the gold standard for LVH).

32. I: NSR 90/min. PR .11, QRS .13, QT normal. Axis 15°. Abnormal due to pre-
excitation (Wolff-Parkinson-White syndrome [WPW]).

C: The PR is borderline short (depends on the lead). There is a delta wave (lead I
or the V leads). Compare this tracing with those demonstrating bundle branch
block. With WPW, the *initial* portion of the QRS is slurred. With BBB, the *terminal*
part of the QRS is slurred. This makes sense when you think of the pathophysiology
of the two conditions (see text). A blocked bundle branch causes a portion of the
heart to be depolarized late, affecting the end of the QRS. There is a tall R wave
in V_1 (consistent with posterior MI), and there are possible Q waves in inferior leads.
Delta waves may appear as pseudo-Q's.

33. I: SVT 180/min. QRS .07, QT long for the rate. Axis 90°. Abnormal due to SVT.
High QRS voltage noted.

C: P waves are not easily seen, although the notched upstroke of the T wave in
the precordial leads could be a P. Atrial flutter is unlikely at a rate of 180/min. With
flutter, the atrial rate is usually 300/min, and the ventricular rate is 1/2, 1/3, or 1/4
of that (with 2:1, 3:1, or 4:1 block). It is not rapid atrial fibrillation, as the rhythm
is regular. This could be a reentrant SVT due to a pre-excitation syndrome; you
would not expect to see delta waves during SVT where antegrade conduction is
through the AV node, right? (See Fig 1.15.)

   When reading the ECG, making the simple diagnosis of SVT is adequate. Most
of these cases are due to AV nodal reentry (the reentrant focus is in the AV node).

34. I: NSR 75/min. PR .22, QRS .08, QT normal. Axis −30°. Abnormal due to first-
degree AV block, LAD, and NSST-TCs.

C: I agree that there is ST elevation in V_2, but not enough to make a diagnosis of
acute ischemia. Also, the ST's have normal upward convexity. There is T inversion,
but it is not the deep, symmetrical T inversion typical of non-Q MI (see ECG No.
27). So I am calling the ST-T changes nonspecific.

   If the pain sounds like angina, treat her with nitroglycerine and aspirin. It would
be important to *repeat the ECG* in 10 to 15 min, especially if the quality or intensity
of pain changes. You might discover increased ST elevation if this is an MI. Finding

an old tracing for comparison would help. In the absence of the marked ST elevation that is typical of acute, transmural MI, I would not recommend thrombolytic therapy. Remember that the risk of intracranial bleeding with thrombolysis is higher for elderly patients.

35. I: AV sequential pacemaker with 100% capture, 60/min.

C: There are pacing spikes before the P wave and QRS. The QRS has an LBBB pattern indicating a right ventricular location of the pacing electrode. This dual-chamber pacemaker, with leads in the right atrium and right ventricle, is called a DDD pacemaker: it has dual-chamber sensing, dual-chamber pacing, and dual sensing modes (pacing that can be either inhibited or triggered by preceding beats).

36. I: NSR 90/min. PR .20, QRS .16, QTc .54. Axis −60°. Abnormal due to RBBB + LAFB, and LVH. Cannot exclude lateral MI of uncertain age.

C: QTc prolongation loses its usual significance when there is bundle branch block (which must alter the sequence of ventricular repolarization as well as depolarization). It is possible to diagnose ventricular hypertrophy and infarction in the presence of RBBB, but not with LBBB. The deep Q in aVL raises the possibility of lateral MI.

LVH indicates that her hypertension has not been adequately controlled. Confirm the diagnosis with an echocardiogram and choose antihypertensive therapy that has been shown to induce regression of hypertrophy (ACE inhibitors and beta-blockers).

37. I: AF 80/min. QRS .10, QT normal. Axis 60°. Abnormal due to AF, anterior MI of uncertain age, and NSST-TCs.

C: The ST-T changes in precordial leads may be related to the old MI. ST sagging in inferior leads looks like digitalis effect (and you would expect that she is taking it as there is AF with good control of the ventricular rate).

38. I: Complete heart block, 36/min. QRS .18, QT normal. Axis 130°. Abnormal due to the complete heart block and a ventricular escape rhythm.

C: At first glance, I called this 2:1 AV block. With the Marquette equipment, the lead changes are instantaneous, and the top line of recording can be read as a continuous rhythm strip. Notice that the P waves that appear to be conducted (every-other P wave) are followed by progressively longer PR intervals. The second-to-last beat has such a long PR that it is hard to believe the P is conducted. And the last beat has a short PR. Despite this variability of the PR, the ventricular rate is constant. The ventricular rate is not a multiple of the atrial rate; but it is close and for this reason has the appearance of 2:1 block. This is an example of AV dissociation and complete heart block.

The ventricular escape rhythm has a rate of 36 beats/min. This relatively rapid rhythm accounts for the absence of syncope. Why not diagnose RBBB + LPFB?

The ventricular beats have that morphology, but they originate from the ventricle. The term *bundle branch block* indicates that the beat originates from above the bundle branch.

39. I: NSR 90/min. PR .16, QRS .90, QT long for the rate. Axis 60°. Abnormal due to acute anterolateral MI and long QT.

C: Acute ischemia is one cause of QT interval prolongation, and patients who have a long QT during their acute MI have an increased risk of ventricular arrhythmias.

There is reciprocal ST depression in inferior leads, but the main event is clearly the anterolateral ST elevation. He already has Q waves in precordial leads, but that does not mean that the MI occurred in the distant past. According to the history he had 2 hours of pain, then relief. It sounds like occlusion of the anterior descending artery, then spontaneous thrombolysis with relief of pain. With reperfusion early in the course of MI, Q waves may evolve rapidly, within minutes. When pain redeveloped, the ST's re-elevated and the Q's remained. Because there is ischemic pain and ST elevation, he must have live muscle in the region, and reperfusion therapy is indicated (recombinant tissue plasminogen activator [rT-PA] or angioplasty).

Anterior infarct size is proportional to the number of leads with ST elevation; in this case V_2 through V_6 plus I and aVL. This is a big MI.

40. I: NSR 60/min. PR .16, QRS .08, QT normal for the rate. Axis 60°. Abnormal due to anterolateral MI. Compared with the prior tracing, ST changes are less prominent and the QT interval is shorter.

C: It appears that thrombolytic therapy was successful. This ECG was done 4 hours later, and there is less ST elevation. The reciprocal ST depression in inferior leads has resolved. Some persistence of ST elevation is typical after successful thrombolysis. Shortening of the QTc from .44 to .40 sec is interesting. It is common to see resolution of conduction abnormalities when infarction is interrupted with thrombolytic therapy. There is a similar beneficial effect of reperfusion on prolonged QT.

41. I: NSR 60/min. PR .18, QRS .09, QT normal. Axis 45°. Borderline ECG due to incomplete RBBB.

C: This may be a normal finding. But IRBBB may indicate RV volume overload (it is a sensitive but not specific finding). For an asymptomatic young person, atrial septal defect (ASD) should be excluded. An echocardiogram would do that. The chest x-ray shows shunt vascularity with ASD. But my first diagnostic study would be a physical exam (fixed splitting of the second heart sound and a soft systolic murmur). If the exam is abnormal, I would order an echo.

42. I: NSR 65/min. PR .16, QRS .10, QT normal. Axis −70°. Abnormal due to IRBBB, LAFB, and PRWP.

C: LAFB is a common cause of PRWP across precordial leads. Here is another case of IRBBB, this time with associated LAFB. There are physical findings to indicate ASD.

The ECG allows you to differentiate primum from secundum ASD. The ostium secundum defect accounts for 85% of ASD's; it affects the superior part of the septum and has no effect on the infranodal conduction system. The primum defect is an abnormality of the endocardial cushion, which also is the origin of the mitral and/or tricuspid valves and the upper part of the interventricular septum, including parts of the infranodal conducting system. Primum ASD's usually affect the anterior fascicle; LAFB thus points to a primum ASD (and a normal axis, to secundum ASD).

The loud murmur probably is mitral regurgitation; with primum defects, there may be a cleft mitral leaflet. The usual systolic murmur of a secundum ASD is soft and is caused by increased flow across a normal pulmonic valve.

43. I: NSR 90/min. PR .18, QRS .09, QT is long for the rate with QTc .54. Axis 70°. Abnormal due to long QT and LAA.

C: There is notching of the P in lead II. The dominant finding is the long QT. Phenothiazine derivatives, including antihistamines, may lengthen the QT interval. When some antihistamines are combined with erythromycin, the QT interval prolongation may be aggravated; this combination may precipitate ventricular arrhythmias. The history of syncope and this ECG are indications for monitoring in the telemetry unit.

44. I: Polymorphic ventricular tachycardia, torsade de pointes.

C: Torsade de pointes is a form of VT that tends to occur with *conditions that prolong the QT interval* (see Table 2.5). Treatment of the arrhythmia includes measures that shorten the QT: magnesium infusion, increasing the heart rate with temporary pacing, or even isoproterenol infusion.

*45. I: **Top:** NSR, 65/min with 3-beat bursts of VT. **Middle:** Monomorphic VT, 170/ min. **Bottom:** Ventricular fibrillation.*

C: Sudden cardiac death from ventricular fibrillation is a common complication of severe LV dysfunction. This patient was resuscitated and subsequently received an implantable defibrillator.

46. I: NSR 85/min with an AV sequential pacemaker and ventricular pacing.

C: There is a P before each QRS. The pacer senses the P wave and paces the ventricle after a pre-set AV (or PR) interval. As the ventricular lead is positioned in the RV, the QRS has an LBBB pattern. Pacing spikes are often small and may not be apparent in all ECG leads.

47. I: Sinus bradycardia (SB) 50/min. PR .14, QRS .08, QT normal. Axis 45°. Abnormal due to T inversion consistent with anterolateral ischemia or non-Q infarction.

C: The deep and symmetrically inverted T's are typical for non-Q infarction (to differentiate that from unstable angina with the same ECG findings depends on cardiac enzymes). In V_2 and V_3, there is a hint of ST elevation. These ST's have slight upward convexity. I am not sure it means anything in the absence of chest pain, but if he had recurrence of pain I would repeat the ECG promptly, looking for more ST elevation. This may be a case for early angiography.

48. I: NSR 95/min. PR .12, QRS .10, QT normal. Axis 45°. Abnormal due to ST elevation, possibly inferolateral ischemia or MI.

C: The ST elevation in inferior leads plus V₅ and V₆ is subtle but definite. There is also reciprocal ST depression in V₁ through V₃. Having an old tracing for comparison would help, but this is probably acute MI. Is it a large or small MI? Recall that with inferior MI, infarct size is proportional to the amount of ST elevation in inferior leads. These ST's are not up very much. The ECG should be repeated in a few minutes, as the degree of ST elevation can vary during the acute MI. It probably is a small MI, and this would figure in decisions about how aggressively to treat. Acute angioplasty has low risk but is not always available. Thrombolytic therapy carries a small but definite risk of intracranial bleeding, and some authorities would recommend avoiding it with small, low-risk MI. This patient has had chest pain for 9 hours, and the chances of salvaging muscle are diminished that late in the course of MI. In the absence of other clinical indicators of high risk with this infarction, I probably would not treat her with thrombolytic agents.

It is important to recognize that ST elevation may be subtle with acute MI. Even with small infarction, there is a risk of early arrhythmias. This patient should be in the hospital on a monitor (not at home taking antacids).

49. I: NSR 95/min. PR .20, QRS .08, QT normal. Axis −30°. Abnormal due to first-degree AV block, LAD, PRWP, NSST-TCs.

C: The PR is borderline. There are small R waves in V₂ and V₃, and this is not an anterior MI. Delayed R progression is probably related to the axis. Note that this ECG report, like many, is descriptive and provides no clinical diagnosis. She has diabetes. Could the T inversion in aVL be a subtle indicator of silent, occult ischemic heart disease? Sure; but that is not an issue to be addressed when reading the ECG.

50. I: SB 50/min. PR .24, QRS .10, QT long for the rate with QTc .57. Axis 70°. Abnormal due to SB, LAA, 1°AV block, long QT, and NSST-TCs.

C: The computer read a possible anterior MI: I see positive glitches at the beginning of the QRS in V₂ and V₃. In this case, with the rate less than 60/min, the QTc is less than the measured QT (recheck Bazett's formula). The ST sagging in V₅ looks like digitalis effect, a good possibility in an elderly man with bradycardia and 1°AV block.

51. I: AF 70/min. QRS .11, QT normal. Axis −50°. Abnormal due to AF, LAFB, NSST-TCs, and PRWP (cannot exclude prior anterior MI or LVH).

C: The premature beat in V₁ could be a PVC, but it may also be a supraventricular beat that is aberrantly conducted. The fact that its axis is similar to those of other beats supports aberrancy. The diagnosis of AF may be incorrect; the first RR intervals in I, aVR, and V_4 are identical. Perhaps it is sinus rhythm with low voltage P's, or a nodal rhythm. But with a rhythm this irregular, I am willing to call it AF (and possibly be wrong). There could be an anterior MI, as just some of the complexes in V_2 and V_3 have small initial R waves. LVH is possible as well: LAD, wide QRS, lateral ST-T changes (see Table 2.1).

There is a lot going on in this ECG. When there are multiple abnormalities, just look at each of the things on your list one at a time (see Table 1.1) and note the findings in your interpretation. It is like caring for a patient in the ICU with multiple problems; it is easiest to have a problem list and deal with each problem individually.

52. I: NSR 80/min. PR .14, QRS .08, QT normal. Axis 70°. Normal ECG.

C: I needed a breather. After looking at a series of abnormal tracings, do you find that a normal seems to jump out at you?

53. I: NSR 70/min, PR .16, QRS .08, QT normal. Axis −40°. Abnormal due to LAD, PRWP, and NSST-TCs.

C: This man has idiopathic, dilated cardiomyopathy, which may account for the relatively low voltage as well as all of the abnormal findings. But there is nothing on the ECG that is specific for cardiomyopathy. The absence of Q waves makes ischemic cardiomyopathy unlikely.

54. I: NSR 80/min. PR .16, QRS .10, QT normal. Axis 30°. Abnormal due to NSST-TCs. Small inferior Q's noted.

C: The small Q's in II and aVF are not enough to call this an inferior MI, despite the history of MI. It is not unusual for the Q's of small inferior infarction to disappear with time. (The most famous example of this was Lyndon Johnson, who carried a miniature of his ECG so that he could show doctors he met and challenge them to find his MI. Recall that he also enjoyed showing his cholecystectomy scar.)

The sagging ST segments suggest digitalis effect; with her history of AF, she may be taking digoxin. Is the QT long? It is hard to be sure.

55. I: NSR 60/min. PR .14, QRS .10, QT normal. Abnormal due to NSST-TCs and small inferior Q's. U wave noted.

C: The U wave is seen in V_2 through V_4; the QTU interval is still in the normal range. Although the Q waves are small, this probably is an inferior MI, because there is associated T inversion in leads III and aVF.

56. I: NSR 70/min. PR .14, QRS .15, QT normal. Axis −50°. Abnormal due to LAA, LAFB, IVCD, PRWP, and NSST-TCs.

C: At first glance, this looks like LBBB; the QRS is wide and terminal forces are aimed to the left. The small Q's in I and aVL—the so-called septal Q's—prevent that diagnosis (see text and Fig 2.4). Because the diagnosis is IVCD rather than LBBB, I mention ST-T changes, delayed R progression, and LAFB in the ECG report.

Because it is not LBBB, why not call it LVH—there are enough criteria (see Table 2.1). Because the conduction abnormality could cause all these findings, I elected not to make that call. It would not be wrong to indicate possible LVH. Infranodal conduction abnormalities are common among elderly patients.

57. I: NSR 95/min. PR .20, QRS .14, QTc .70. Axis −40°. Abnormal due to LAA, LBBB, and a long QT interval.

C: LAA may be a reach, but I think the P is broad and notched in III, and roughly biphasic in V₁. LBBB may be responsible for long QT; QT prolongation does not have the same significance in the presence of gross conduction abnormalities. But this QT is so impressive that I decided to mention it, particularly as there is a history of arrhythmia. At the least, he should have his electrolytes checked and medicines reviewed.

58. I: NSR 60/min. PR .14, QRS .09, QT normal. Axis −60°. Abnormal due to LAD plus inferolateral MI of uncertain age, NSST-TCs.

C: Because of inferior Q waves, call this LAD rather than LAFB. The Q waves are impressive; I elected to call them inferolateral rather than inferior + lateral or inferior + anterior.

The patient had no history of MI. An echocardiogram showed marked thickening of the interventricular septum plus other features of idiopathic hypertrophic subaortic stenosis (IHSS), a form of hypertrophic cardiomyopathy. We tend to think of Q waves as specific for myocardial scar; it is a reliable finding, as exceptions (false positives) are uncommon. IHSS and WPW can fool you with a pseudoinfarct pattern.

59. I: NSR 90/min. PR .15, QRS .07, QT normal. Axis 120°. Abnormal due to LAA, RAD, probable RVH with associated repolarization changes.

C: The relatively low voltage is typical of emphysema. RAD, the tall R in V₁ and deep S in V₆ (relative to overall voltage), plus the T changes in right precordial leads make RVH likely. She has cor pulmonale. Note that her LAA is an unrelated finding, not a part of the RVH or cor pulmonale syndrome. You might expect to see RAA, not LAA.

60. I: ST 110/min. PR .14, QRS .08, QT normal. Axis −35°. Abnormal due to ST, LAD, probable LAA, and anterior MI of uncertain age.

C: Sinus tachycardia at rest is consistent with his known congestive heart failure and suggests LV decompensation. LAA is consistent with increased pulmonary capillary wedge pressure. There are Q's in just three precordial leads, changes that are not that extensive. Infarction patterns on the ECG do not always reflect the degree of cardiac disability. Perhaps he has hypertensive heart disease or cardiomyopathy in addition to his ischemic heart disease. Again, the resting tachycardia may be the most telling finding.

61. I: Atrial flutter with 2:1 block, 130/min. QRS .14, QT long for the rate. Axis 60°.

Abnormal due to rhythm, unusual P axis, RBBB and associated repolarization changes, possible inferolateral MI of uncertain age.

C: The ventricular rate in atrial flutter with 2:1 block is usually 150/min. But there appear to be flutter waves in lead II. The inferolateral Q's are small but worth mention. ST depression may all be due to RBBB, but it could reflect ischemia in a patient with chest pain. We are not given that history. Comparison of this with a prior ECG is important, particularly for an acutely ill patient.

62. I: Atrial fibrillation 90/min. QRS .10, QT normal. Axis −10°. Abnormal due to rhythm, NSST-TCs.

C: There appear to be flutter waves in inferior leads. This could be called atrial flutter with variable block, or atrial flutter-fib. Because atrial flutter is usually a regular rhythm, and I find no area where the rhythm is regular, I have called this AF. But you can see where there may be some blending of the two conditions. It looks like the T's are inverted in inferior leads and flat in V_5 and V_6, but these apparent changes may be due to the flutter waves.

As a rule, patients with AF need anticoagulation (to prevent peripheral embolism), and those with atrial flutter do not. Based on this ECG, I cannot be sure about the status of atrial contraction and would treat him with warfarin. The trials of anticoagulation for AF generally identified elderly patients as having the highest risk for peripheral embolism.

63. I: NSR 90/min. PR .20, QRS .12, QT normal. Axis 60°. Abnormal due to RBBB and acute anterolateral MI.

C: Axis—the QRS looks most isoelectric in aVL, and it is positive in II. The QRS is wide enough for bundle branch block. Rather than an RSR pattern in V_1, there is a qR pattern; the initial positive deflection is lost because of the anterior MI.

This is another unusual ECG in which ST elevation involves multiple vascular regions. I believe it is infarction rather than pericarditis for a few reasons: the degree of ST elevation (I have never seen pericarditis push the ST's this high), the upward convexity of ST's, the early T inversion in V_2, the associated Q waves, and the patient's age (acute pericarditis is more commonly an illness of younger patients, and this man is in the coronary age group). He probably has a substantial anterior descending artery with large branches that reach the lateral wall.

It is a big MI. Recall that the size of anterior MI is proportional to the number of leads with ST elevation, not the degree of elevation. I count nine leads with elevated ST's. Once, an elderly man who had had coronary artery spasm, ST elevation, and terrible chest pain told me later, "Doc, that was the Big Mac." Well, this looks like the Big Mac to me. This man needs urgent reperfusion therapy.

64. I: ST 100/min. PR .24, QRS .10, QT normal. Axis 10°. Abnormal due to 1°AV block and NSST-TCs. Small inferior Q's noted.

C: In a couple of leads (II, V_4), it appears that the QT is long. But in leads where the P and the T waves are distinct (V_2 and V_3), it is apparent that the P is making the end of the T wave difficult to see. There seems to be a small initial R wave in III, and the small, isolated Q in aVF does not make the diagnosis of MI. I decided to call the flat and slightly depressed STs in V$_2$ through V$_4$ abnormal; if that had been the only abnormality, I probably would not have done so.

Consider digitalis toxicity with the long PR interval, confusion, and blurred vision.

65. I: NSR 70/min. PR .22, QRS .14, QT normal. Axis −60°. Abnormal due to 1°AV block, LAFB, IVCD, NSST-TCs, and PRWP.

C: It is not LBBB because of the septal Q (aVL). The PRWP may be the result of the conduction abnormality, but it could reflect anterior injury (look at the ST and T changes). Nevertheless, delayed R progression is a nonspecific finding, and speculation about possible infarction is the role of the patient's doctor, not the ECG reader. In the presence of conduction disease like this, a false positive stress test is a possibility. An exercise perfusion scan or exercise echocardiogram would be better.

66. I: NSR, 90/min. PR .08, QRS .14, QT normal. Axis −60°. Abnormal due to pre-excitation.

C: It looks like LBBB, but the short PR and the patient's age raise the possibility of WPW—that was my diagnosis. In a number of leads, the delta wave slurs the up-stroke of the QRS, and the terminal portion of the QRS looks normal. Interventricular conduction abnormalities tend to slur the tail end of the QRS (see ECG No. 65).

The next day, her ECG looked normal. Conduction through the bypass tract may come and go. Bundle branch block seldom varies.

67. I: AF 50/min. QRS .14, QT normal. Axis −50°. Abnormal due to AF with slow ventricular response, IVCD, PRWP, and inferolateral MI of uncertain age.

C: This 86-year-old patient is not taking digoxin. His slow ventricular rate with AF indicates a sick AV node. His symptoms indicate that he may be having more severe bradyarrhythmias. I would admit him to a telemetry bed, expecting to document long pauses. He would then receive a pacemaker. Why not get an outpatient, ambulatory monitor? With symptoms for just 1 week and this ECG, I am concerned about syncope and injury.

68. I: Probable wandering atrial pacemaker 90/min (suggest rhythm strip). PR variable, QRS .08, QT normal. Axis 55°. Abnormal due to rhythm, NSST-TCs.

C: An alternative to wandering atrial pacemaker would be NSR with PAC's. The rhythm could be due to digitalis toxicity, but it is as likely related to her age. The ST's are sagging in precordial leads; I would at least check a digoxin level.

69. I: NSR 75/min. PR .13, QRS .08, QT normal. Axis 90°. Borderline due to tall peaked T's consistent with hyperkalemia; may be a normal variant.

C: This patient was taking hydrochlorothiazide and spironolactone, plus KCl. Her potassium was 5.8. When the potassium was stopped, her T wave amplitude fell.

The T wave changes in this ECG are typical of mild hyperkalemia. With higher potassium, the T's get much taller, and T wave amplitude can exceed that of the QRS. (A student once told me he imagined numerous small K's under the tall T wave.) Conduction abnormalities then appear (wider QRS, prolonged PR). With hyperkalemia, bradyarrhythmias (heart block) are the rule; hypokalemia may precipitate ventricular ectopic rhythms.

70. I: Wide-complex tachycardia 140/min, possibly ventricular tachycardia. QRS .20, QT long for the rate. Axis −80°. Abnormal due to rhythm, LBBB pattern. Clinical correlation needed.

C: This is another tracing where I am unsure about the rhythm. The LBBB pattern favors VT, whereas RBBB would suggest aberrant conduction and SVT. The glitch at the beginning of the QRS in II and aVF could be a P wave, suggesting a supraventricular rhythm of some sort (possibly nodal tachycardia with a retrograde P). But it is impossible to tell from this tracing. In addition to hedging, it seems best, to me, to indicate the most serious possibility in the ECG report.

   If the patient is stable, recording bigger P's with an esophageal or right atrial lead would provide an answer. If unstable, DC cardioversion would be justified. With such an arrhythmia, you should measure electrolytes (including magnesium) and a digoxin level.

71. I: Atrial pacemaker, 100% capture at 100/min. QRS .08, QT long for the rate. Axis 30°. Abnormal due to pacer, low QRS voltage, inferolateral ischemia, possibly acute MI.

C: These pacing spikes look different from others you have seen; they have high amplitude, are biphasic, and have a slowly tailing end that makes them look like QRS complexes. However, they are followed by low-voltage QRS's that in turn are followed by T waves. These pacing spikes are typical of *unipolar* leads. *Bipolar* leads have lower amplitude, are sharper, and tend to be uniphasic (see ECG No. 35). Pacing the atrium has no effect on QRS morphology, and it is possible to diagnose ischemia with inferolateral ST elevation plus reciprocal ST depression in anterior leads.

72. I: ST 120/min. PR .16, QRS .14, QT long for the rate. Axis −20°. Abnormal due to rate and LBBB, not present on the prior ECG.

C: This may be rate-related bundle branch block. The LBBB could resolve when the heart rate comes down. No specific treatment is needed other than a repeat ECG. Could the conduction change indicate intraoperative MI? That is a possibility, but the odds are against it with no prior history of coronary disease. Overnight observation on a monitor and cardiac enzymes would be sensible. Consider an echocardiogram (regional wall motion changes).

73. I: NSR 75/min. PR .22, QRS .08, QT long for the rate with QTc .48. Axis 60°. Abnormal due to 1° AV block, long QT, and NSST-TCs.

C: The QT interval is borderline. I thought there might be a U wave tacked on the end of the T in V₂ and made the call. I may be wrong. The sagging ST's could be digitalis effect; especially in a patient with a long PR.

74. I: NSR 90/min. PR .14, QRS .09, QT normal. Axis 30°. Abnormal due to acute inferior ischemia, possibly MI, and PRWP.

C: This could be an inferolateral MI as there is slight ST elevation in V₆ as well as the inferior leads. The degree of ST elevation is minimal, so this is not a large inferior infarction. On the other hand, there are reciprocal ST-T changes in anterior leads plus I and aVL. I think she meets criteria for reperfusion therapy, particularly as you are getting to it early in the course of infarction. But if she had a contraindication to thrombolytic therapy, and angioplasty was not available, I would not feel bad for her. It is probably a low-risk MI.

75. I: NSR 95/min with PVC's. PR .14, QRS .08, QT normal. Abnormal due to PVC's, anterior MI of uncertain age.

C: With this ECG, you can be sure that the ectopic beats are ventricular and not atrial with aberrant conduction (even with the RBBB pattern). With calipers or the edge of a piece of paper, measure the normal P to P interval. Now measure from the P wave of the last sinus beat before the ectopic beat in V₁. Just where the next P should arrive, there is a glitch on the upstroke of the ectopic QRS. That glitch probably is a P wave that comes on time and is not conducted. The subsequent P wave also comes on time, so that the atrial rhythm is not reset by the ectopic beat. This is an example of AV dissociation. As the ectopic does not affect the atria, it must originate in the ventricle.

76. I: Uncertain rhythm, no P waves seen, 75/min. QRS .09, QT normal. Axis 110°. Abnormal due to rhythm, RAD, low voltage, and RVH.

C: This could be atrial flutter; look at the baseline in V₁ for possible flutter waves. The rate is right for 4:1 conduction, and flutter is common with obstructive lung disease. Another possibility is a nodal rhythm. The diagnosis of RVH is supported by ST-T changes in right and midprecordial leads, in addition to the R in V₁, deep S in V₆, and RAD. She has cor pulmonale.

77. I: NSR 65/min. PR .20, QRS .08, QT normal. Axis 45°. Abnormal due to probable anterior ischemia; possible anterior MI.

C: In addition to T inversion, there is slight ST elevation in anterior leads, more than is usually seen with non-Q MI. Perhaps there is a tiny positive glitch (R wave) in V₂, perhaps not. Creatine kinase rose (to twice normal), consistent with non-Q MI.

78. I: SB 58/min. PR .12, QRS .10, QT normal. Axis 45°. Abnormal due to acute inferior MI with reciprocal ST depression in lateral leads.

C: A young person with his first MI. Do not waste any time. Treat him with tissue plasminogen activator. By the time you can get an ambulance and have him transferred to a catheterization lab—at least 2 hours and probably longer in my experience—the infarct artery could be open.

79. I: NSR 70/min. PR .12, QRS .09, QT normal. Abnormal due to ST-T changes consistent with inferolateral ischemia. Since the prior ECG, there is less ST elevation.

C: While the ST segments have come down considerably, there is still some elevation. That is often the case after successful thrombolysis. There is disagreement about what to do at this stage. Many believe that a few days of anticoagulation, then long-term aspirin and beta blocker therapy, are adequate. My colleagues and I feel that angiography and possibly a revascularization procedure are needed because of the high risk of reocclusion. I suspect that is the majority opinion in the cardiology community; but a standard of care after thrombolysis has not been established.

80. I: ST 120/min, PR .12, QRS .10, QT long for the rate with QTc .46. Abnormal due to ST and acute inferior ischemia. Compared with the prior ECG, ST elevation in III and in aVF may be more prominent.

C: He probably has reoccluded. As he remained in the small community hospital, immediate angiography and angioplasty were unavailable. Now the choices are re-treatment with rT-PA, emergency transfer for rescue angioplasty, or traditional measures for acute MI. I am not excited about further thrombolytic therapy; the ST segments are not dramatically higher than before, and the pain could be postinfarction pericarditis (with thrombolytic drugs, there may be a risk of bleeding into the pericardium). With early angiography after thrombolytic therapy, he probably would have avoided this uncertain and unstable situation.

81. I: NSR 65/min. PR .12, QRS .08, QT long for the rate with QTc .56. Axis indeterminant. Abnormal due to posterolateral MI with acute lateral ischemia.

C: The QRS is isoelectric in multiple limb leads; if anything, the QRS vector is pointed back toward lead aVR. The tall R in V_1 is considered the equivalent of a posterior wall Q wave (perhaps you would see a Q if you positioned a V lead on the patient's back). Posterior or posterolateral MI may be caused by occlusion of the circumflex artery (see Fig 2.8). There appears to be active ischemia, with persistent ST elevation and chest pain. An additional finding is tall, peaked T's in V_2 and V_3; these may be the hyperacute T waves of acute ischemia.

The presence of Q waves does not mean that the MI is complete; continued pain and ST elevation just 3 hours from the onset of symptoms are indications for angioplasty or thrombolytic therapy.

82. I: Probably nodal rhythm, 70/min (no P waves seen). QRS .08, QT normal. Axis 0°. Abnormal due to rhythm and NSST-TCs.

C: Regular rhythm with no P's and a narrow QRS complex—probably nodal. Because of the rate, it could be called an accelerated nodal rhythm.

I agree that the regional T inversion in inferolateral leads could be non-Q MI.

Because they are not deep and symmetrically inverted (the usual case with anterior non-Q MI), I am not making that diagnosis. It is a diagnosis the clinician could make if the patient had ischemic chest pain and elevation of cardiac enzymes.

83. I: AF 130/min. QRS .08, QTc .38. Axis 65°. Abnormal due to AF and NSST-TCs.

C: The QT is more than half the RR interval, but the calculated QTc is normal. The ST depression could be ischemic, precipitated by the rapid rate. It would not be wrong to raise that possibility in the ECG report. But there are other possible causes of ST depression such as digoxin or LVH; tachycardia can aggravate ST depression from any cause. I prefer to call the ST-T changes nonspecific, and leave the diagnosis to the clinician. Follow-up: this patient had a pulmonary embolus.

84. I: ST 120/min. PR .18, QRS .10, QT long for the rate (QTc .50). Axis 30°. Abnormal due to acute inferior MI with reciprocal ST depression in anterolateral leads.

C: The ST elevation in the inferior leads is less prominent than the ST depression in anterolateral leads. Nevertheless, ST elevation defines the location of the MI. This patient had occlusion of a large right coronary artery, and the other vessels were normal. The presence of reciprocal ST depression identifies an inferior infarction as a large one. ST elevation and pain indicate transmural ischemia and infarction in progress, usually with (total) occlusion of the coronary artery.

85. I: NSR 80/min. PR .14, QRS .07, QT normal. Probably normal ECG; small inferior Q's noted.

C: The Q's are not deep and wide enough to diagnose MI but are worth mention. Before he starts the new exercise program, he should have a stress test. With the flat ST's in inferolateral leads, the chance of a false positive study may be higher. Combining the exercise ECG with a perfusion scan or echocardiogram would avoid this and provide additional reassurance about the inferior Q's. (The myocardial scar does not take up isotope, nor does it contract.)

86. I: NSR with PVC's, PR .18, QRS .10, QT normal. Abnormal due to LAA. Small inferior Q's noted.

C: Can you be sure these are PVC's? I think so. There are glitches in the ectopic beats in II and III, and in aVL and aVF that are probably P waves; they come on time and have the same axis as the other P's. As the ectopic beat does not reset the sinoatrial pacemaker, there is a *compensatory pause* following the PVC. AV dissociation makes these PVC's, not PAC's with aberrancy.

The P in V$_1$ is biphasic, and it is broad and notched in inferior leads. Even in the absence of other abnormalities, LAA is an important finding in a patient with hypertension. It has been described as the earliest ECG evidence for hypertensive heart disease, appearing much sooner than other signs of LVH. I would be concerned about inadequate control of this patient's hypertension.

87. I: SB 50/min with a burst of wide-complex tachycardia at 150/min, probably ventricular tachycardia. PR .36, QRS .20, QT normal. Axis 30°. Abnormal due to rhythm, 1°AV block, LBBB.

C: Do not let the arrhythmia—a dramatic event admittedly—distract you from reading the rest of the ECG. The paroxysmal tachyarrhythmia looks like VT, but I may be wrong. Without AV dissociation, an atrial arrhythmia with aberrant conduction is always a possibility. In this case, the ventricular rate is 150/min, the typical rate of atrial flutter with 2:1 block. Look at V_2: in the fourth to sixth beats I think you may see flutter waves at 300/min. And in V_4, the last beat is followed by a tiny P that is not conducted. But it still looks like VT to me.

88. I: NSR with ventricular pacing (AV sequential pacer), 95/min. QRS .16, QT long for the rate (QTc .48). Abnormal due to rhythm, RBBB + LAFB pattern.

C: Most pacers that are positioned at the apex of the right ventricle produce an LBBB complex (the RV is depolarized first, the LV last; see Fig 2.4). This wire is pacing the left ventricle; with LAFB, it probably is pacing the left posterior fascicle. There are a few causes of LV pacing: 1) an RV lead may erode through the septum to the LV; 2) the pacing electrode may have been positioned in the coronary sinus (which courses behind the LV); 3) an epicardial electrode could have been screwed into the surface of the LV (as opposed to a transvenous, intracardiac electrode). This can be sorted out with previous ECGs and a chest x-ray. Is there an infarct pattern? With the pacemaker as the origin of the QRS, I would be reluctant to call the inferior Q waves significant, even with the RBBB pattern.

89. I: NSR 70/min. PR .16, QRS .09, QT normal. Axis 15°. Abnormal due to NSST-TCs. Consider inferior ischemia or non-Q MI. U wave noted, and there is QT-U prolongation.

C: Compare this with ECG No. 82. The T in lead III looks more like non-Q MI in this tracing, so I raise that possibility. In the absence of Q's, the diagnosis of MI is rarely made from the ECG alone. It requires ECG, clinical history, and enzyme changes. She needs further evaluation. Start by finding a previous ECG for comparison.

90. I: NSR 90/min. PR .14, QRS .09, QT normal. Axis 20°. Abnormal due to possible anterior MI, and small inferior Q's.

C: I am not sure of the diagnosis of anterior MI. There is a Q in V_5 but in none of the other anterior leads. You would expect V_5 to have an appearance somewhere between that of V_4 and V_6. It could be that the electrode for V_5 was placed an interspace too low on the chest wall. A repeat ECG, or a previous tracing, might show a small R in V_5, indicating that he has PRWP rather than anterior MI.

I have not included many comparisons with prior ECG's in this exercise because of space. Comparison with prior ECG's should always be a part of the ECG report.

91. I: NSR 60/min. PR .18, QRS .16, QT normal. Axis −60°. Abnormal due to RBBB + LAFB, and anterior MI of uncertain age.

C: The small initial R wave in inferior leads makes LAFB more likely than inferior MI. This is another example of our ability to diagnose MI in the presence of RBBB.

92. I: NSR 90/min. PR .14, QRS .08, QT normal. Axis 15°. Abnormal due to NSST-TCs.

C: I see a bit of ST elevation in V₂. I doubt that it means anything, and I would not have called this an abnormal ECG if that was the only finding. In this case, there are T wave changes in inferolateral leads.

93. I: ST 120/min. PR .16, QRS .09, QT normal. Axis 60°. No obvious abnormality, but there is marked baseline artifact; consider repeat ECG.

C: What a mess! But, if you look carefully, you can make a number of observations (note my measurements). I am also confident that there are no Q's or major ST-T changes. This may be electrical artifact—a technical problem with the ECG machine. But it could also be caused by shivering or tremor.

94. I: NSR 60/min. QRS .09, QT normal. Axis 0°. Borderline due to small inferior Q's and possible LAA.

C: Look at how broad and notched the P waves are in leads II and V₂ and V₃, a soft finding. The inferior Q's are borderline. Another abnormality is the early transition in V₂. Posterior MI is one cause of this, but tall R's are usually seen in V₁ as well. He was referred because of the heart attack pattern on his ECG. To sort it out, the choices include exercise perfusion scan, echocardiogram, and cardiac catheterization.

95. I: NSR 70/min. PR .18, QRS .08, QT normal. Axis −30°. Abnormal due to LAD, inferior MI of uncertain age, and NSST-TCs.

C: Compare these Q's with the last patient's.

96. I: Accelerated junctional rhythm 90/min. QRS .10, QT normal for the rate. Axis 30°. Abnormal due to rhythm, possibly acute inferolateral ischemia or MI. Cannot exclude pericarditis. Clinical correlation needed.

C: There are no P waves, the rhythm is regular, and the QRS complexes are narrow. Acute MI may be complicated by a variety of supraventricular arrhythmias (most commonly ST, AF, and rapid nodal rhythms). But pericarditis may provoke supraventricular arrhythmias as well. With reciprocal ST depression, we could be sure that this is an inferior MI; but he does not have it. Another possibility is that the diffuse inferolateral ST elevation is pericarditis.

97. I: SB 55/min. PR .18, QRS .09, QT-U long for the rate. Axis 80°. Probably normal ECG, U wave noted.

C: I calculate the QT-U at .50 in V₂. It may be unimportant, but what if he is taking diuretics? As the long QT-U is the only abnormality, I called this ECG normal.

98. I: NSR 80/min. PR .18, QRS .08, QT normal. Axis 45°. Abnormal due to anterior MI of uncertain age.

C: It is possible that a repeat ECG would document a small initial R in V$_2$, and that the present findings are due to lead placement.

99. I: NSR 70/min. PR .16, QRS .09, QT normal. Axis 45°. Borderline due to IRBBB.

C: As an isolated finding, this is not enough to make the ECG abnormal; most cases of IRBBB are normal variants. But think of conditions that could cause RV volume overload when you see this pattern in one of your patients. In the absence of clinical evidence of RV overload, further diagnostic testing is not necessary.

100. I: NSR 70/min. PR .13, QRS .08, QT normal. Axis −20°. Borderline due to NSST-TCs. Unusual P axis noted.

C: The abnormal P axis indicates that the rhythm does not originate in the SA node; *NSR* is technically incorrect. It is probably a low atrial or coronary sinus pacemaker.

Other possibilities: 1) In some leads the PR looks short, raising the possibility of pre-excitation. But the PR is over 0.12 sec in the inferior leads, and there is no delta wave. 2) These could be retrograde P's that originate in the upper part of the AV node. When such high nodal rhythms cause a P that precedes the QRS, the PR interval is usually shorter than it is in this case. Low atrial rhythms with negative P's in the inferior leads are not considered clinically significant. They point to no structural heart disease and have no clinical consequences.

A potentially noteworthy finding is early transition of the R wave in precordial leads. Posterior MI can do this, but there are usually inferior Q's as well. RVH is another cause, but the tall R should be seen in V$_1$. Lead misplacement is probably the most common cause of early transition.

101. I: NSR 70/min. PR .16, QRS .10, QT normal. Normal ECG.

C: T wave inversion that is limited to V$_1$ or to III is not considered abnormal. Similarly, an isolated Q in III is not abnormal. I suppose that you could comment that small inferior Q's are noted while still calling it a normal ECG. But you do not have to, and you will not be doing him any favor with this insurance exam.

102. I: Blocked PAC's.

C: Look carefully at the T wave that precedes the pause. It is different from the other T's, and the distortion is the ectopic P wave. Blocked PAC's are commonly responsible for pauses and are diagnosed when distortion of the preceding T wave is recognized.

103. I: The rhythm strip shows AV nodal Wenckebach (Mobitz I second-degree block).

C: There is progressive lengthening of the PR before the blocked beat, and the PR that follows the dropped beat is shorter. (Review Fig 1.9.)

104. I: NSR with ventricular bigeminy 90/min. PR .23, QRS .08, QT normal. Axis −40°. Abnormal due to rhythm, 1°AV block, LAD, probable inferior MI of uncertain age.

C: Features that support a diagnosis of PVC's: wide complexes, QRS axis opposite that of the T wave (i.e., upright QRS, inverted T), uniphasic QRS in most leads. Features suggesting PAC's with aberrancy: the initial vector of the ectopic beats is the same as that of normal beats, at least in the precordial leads. Because we cannot see P waves near the ectopic beats (looking for AV dissociation), we cannot be sure. But they look like PVC's to me.

105. I: NSR 90/min. PR .16, QRS .14, QT normal. Axis −70°. Abnormal due to RBBB, LAFB, possible RVH.

C: The conduction abnormality adds uncertainty, but the tall R in V_1 and deep S in V_6 suggest RVH.

106. I: NSR 90/min. PR .16, QRS .09, QT normal. Axis 30°. Borderline ECG due to possible inferior MI of uncertain age. Early repolarization noted.

C: The Q's are borderline. Early repolarization is not considered an abnormality. It is a common finding in thin, young athletes (which this man is not). Roughly 10% to 15% of MIs are clinically silent. This patient needs further evaluation.

107. I: NSR 70/min. PR .14, QRS .08, QT long with QTc .50. Abnormal due to anterior ischemia and possible non-Q MI, and long QT interval.

C: Ischemia is one cause of long QT interval, and patients who have it have a greater risk of VT during acute MI. Thrombolytic therapy is not indicated in the absence of chest pain and ST segment elevation. But he should be anticoagulated and should have angiography.

108. I: NSR 95/min. PR .19, QRS .08, QT borderline for the rate. Axis 10°. Abnormal due to acute inferior MI.

C: Yes; ST elevation indicating transmural infarction is the usual ECG indication for urgent reperfusion (thrombolytic therapy or angioplasty, depending on your setting). The other ECG indication for reperfusion therapy—not present in this case—is new bundle branch block with acute MI. This is a big inferior MI, based on the amount of ST elevation in inferior leads plus reciprocal ST depression in lateral leads.

109. I: Atrial flutter with 4:1 conduction. QRS .09, QT long for the rate (QTc .50). Axis 80°. Abnormal due to rhythm, long QT, and NSST-TCs. Small inferior Q's noted.

C: The voltage in V_5 suggests LVH; it just misses being high enough. Because she is on digoxin, the ST sagging counts less LVH. It looks more like digitalis effect, though a bit deep.

110. I: NSR with nodal Wenckebach and 3:2 conduction. QRS .16, QT normal. Abnormal due to rhythm and LBBB.

C: A rhythm strip would help, but we can make a diagnosis from this tracing. Look at the P waves in aVF. The first complete cycle has a long PR, and the last beat has a much longer PR, then some distortion of the T wave (due to the P wave which comes on time). There is a pause; the next beat (now we are into V₃—this is a continuous tracing), has a short PR.

I have told you that you cannot diagnose acute MI in the presence of LBBB, but this may be an exception. The ST elevation in III and aVF is suggestive. Wencke-bach is a common arrhythmia with inferior MI (see ECG No. 103), and the patient is having chest pain. Because of bundle branch block and this clinical presentation, she had immediate catheterization which showed an occluded right coronary artery. This was opened with angioplasty.

111. I: SB 55/min. PR .14, QRS .14, QT normal. Abnormal due to LBBB. Since the prior ECG, heart block and inferior ST elevation have resolved and there is new T inversion.

C: This follow-up tracing allows us to be sure that acute MI was the illness at presentation. Her doctor was right to give her reperfusion therapy. There was a subsequent, small rise in cardiac enzymes.

Conduction abnormalities caused by acute MI tend to resolve promptly with successful reperfusion therapy. That was the case with her AV nodal block. The fact that the LBBB did not resolve suggests that it was an old problem.

112. I: ST 100/min. PR .15, QRS .09, QT normal. Axis 0°. Abnormal due to biatrial enlargement and LVH with repolarization changes.

C: There is a tall P in II (arguable) in addition to the biphasic P in V₁. LVH: voltage, LAA, and lateral ST-T changes.

113. I: ST 100/min. PR .20, QRS .10, QT borderline (QTc .45). Axis −45°. Abnormal due to LAD, anterior and inferior MI of uncertain age.

C: I do not usually diagnose LAFB when there are inferior Q's; instead, I indicate left axis deviation. This patient has had two MI's. Neither was treated with reperfusion therapy, and he now has ischemic cardiomyopathy. Patients with this diagnosis have a history of MI and/or Q waves on the ECG. By contrast, those with idiopathic, dilated cardiomyopathy usually do not have Q waves or a clinical history of MI.

114. I: AF 160/min. QRS .07, QTc .47. Axis 70°. Abnormal due to AF and a rapid ventricular response, and NSST-TCs.

C: The ST-T changes probably are rate related, but I cannot exclude active ischemia. She probably has paroxysmal AF; rule out anemia and hyperthyroidism, and get an echocardiogram to assess left atrial size and LV function, and to screen for other structural abnormalities.

115. I: ST with PAC's, 120/min. PR .12, QRS .16, QTc .50. Abnormal due to long QT, RBBB, ST elevation consistent with acute anterior ischemia or MI.

C: She has the clinical syndrome of MI with two ECG indications for reperfusion therapy: bundle branch block (possibly new) and ST segment elevation. Multicenter trials have shown that thrombolytic therapy improves the survival of elderly patients with MI.

116. I: NSR 80/min. PR .14, QRS .08, QTc .50. Abnormal due to QT interval prolongation.

C: You have looked at a number of ECGs with borderline QT prolongation. This seems frequently the case when the underlying rhythm is fast. The QT prolongation on this ECG is the real thing. Both phenothiazines and tricyclic antidepressants may cause QT prolongation.

117. I: ST 120/min. PR .14, QRS .09, QT normal for the rate. Axis 120°. Abnormal due to RVH.

C: This young woman probably has Eisenmenger's syndrome. In addition to a murmur, I would expect to find clubbing of her fingers and a right ventricular heave. Lethargy may be due to polycythemia.

118. I: NSR 75/min. PR .12, QRS .09, QT normal. Axis 60°. Abnormal due to biatrial abnormality and LVH with repolarization changes.

C: I count 6 points for LVH: LAA plus ST-T changes. Voltage just misses (see Table 2.1).

119. I: AF 60 to 70/min. QRS .10, QT normal. Axis 20°. Abnormal due to rhythm, NSST-TCs, and possible LVH.

C: There is high voltage, but no other criterion for LVH. This is a good example of J-point depression with upsloping ST's (lead V$_6$). He has Marfan's syndrome and aortic regurgitation. An echocardiogram showed that the LV was dilated but not thickened.

120. I: Probable junctional bradycardia (no P's seen). QRS .09, QT normal. Axis 45°. Abnormal due to rhythm, NSST-TCs and PRWP (cannot exclude anterior MI).

C: I cannot be sure about retrograde P's, although they may account for the glitch at the end of the QRS in I, II, aVL, and V$_2$ through V$_4$. Even without retrograde P's, nodal rhythm is the diagnosis when there are no P's, the QRS is narrow, and the rhythm is regular. There is a small initial R wave in V$_2$ through V$_4$ making anterior MI less likely. But one of the causes of PRWP is anterior MI; mentioning that possibility is not an error.

121. I: NSR 85/min. PR .20, QRS .14, QT normal. Axis −60°. Abnormal due to RBBB + LAFB, ST elevation indicating acute anterior ischemia, probably MI.

C: You can diagnose acute infarction in the presence of RBBB. It seems, at first glance, that ST elevation is limited to V$_2$, but there probably is elevation in V$_1$ and V$_3$ as well. Reperfusion therapy is not too late 6 hours after the onset of MI; some studies have shown benefit even at 12 hours.

122. I: NSR 80/min. PR .14, QRS .14, QT long for the rate (QTc .50). Axis −60°. Abnormal due to LBBB.

C: Why not LVH? He has LAD, ST-T changes, possible LAA, and nearly voltage criteria. But with LBBB, we are not able to make that diagnosis. The conduction abnormality itself may cause these changes. The clinical issue is whether the patient has hypertensive heart disease. LBBB generally occurs in a setting of organic heart disease, and there is a history of hypertension. Hypertensive heart disease is likely, and an echocardiogram would help to sort it out.

123. I: NSR 70/min. PR .20, QRS .11, QT normal. Axis −60°. Abnormal due to LAFB and PRWP.

C: There are small initial R waves in III and aVF; I do not think he has inferior Q's. This is a common cardiology consult. The issue can be settled with an echo or a perfusion scan. Poor R wave progression commonly accompanies LAFB.

124. I: NSR 65/min. PR .18, QRS .10, QT normal. Axis 70°. Abnormal due to acute inferior ischemia, probable MI.

C: It is a small MI given the magnitude of ST elevation. On the other hand, there is reciprocal ST depression (V_2 and aVL). Should she be treated? It is a borderline case. I would probably not use thrombolytic therapy; her age increases the risk of intracranial bleeding, and this looks like a small (low-risk) MI. There are plenty of reasonable people in the business who would not hesitate to take her directly to the catheterization lab, or even to try thrombolysis. A lot depends on other clinical circumstances and how she feels about treatment.

125. I: NSR 75/min. PR .20, QRS .10, QT long (QTc .54). Axis 45°. Abnormal due to long QT and NSST-TCs.

C: This QT interval is clearly longer than half the RR interval. I do not usually call the borderline cases where the QT is just at half the RR. She may be on thiazides (check electrolytes including magnesium). She may also be taking an antiarrhythmic agent that prolongs the QT, such as quinidine, which may be used to treat paroxysmal AF.

126. I: Multifocal atrial tachycardia (MAT), 130/min. PR variable. QRS .08, QT normal. Axis −30°. Abnormal due to rhythm, LAD, and low QRS voltage.

C: MAT most commonly occurs in patients with obstructive lung disease. Verapamil is the first choice for control of the ventricular rate. Digoxin may also be used, but beware of digitalis toxicity, as patients with obstructive lung disease seem especially sensitive to the drug.

127. I: Nodal bradycardia, 50/min. QRS .10, QT normal. Axis 20°. Abnormal due to the rhythm and inferior ST elevation; cannot exclude ischemia.

C: The sharp glitch just beyond the peak of the T wave in leads II, III, and aVF looks like a retrograde P wave. ST changes after heart surgery are difficult to interpret. They are usually caused by surgery-induced pericarditis; many patients have a pericardial friction rub during the few days after surgery. In this case, the isolated changes in inferior leads appear ischemic.

128. I: NSR 80/min. PR .16, QRS .08, QT normal. Axis 45°. Abnormal due to lateral ischemia, probably acute lateral MI.

C: ST elevation is limited to leads I and aVL and V$_{4-6}$, and there are reciprocal changes (ST depression) in inferior leads.

129. I: NSR 90/min with PVC's. PR .16, QRS .10, QT normal. Axis−50°. Abnormal due to LAA, LAFB, anterior MI of uncertain age.

C: There is a P wave at the end of the premature beat in I and II; the ectopic beat does not reset the atrial rhythm. AV dissociation identifies the ectopic beat as ventricular. LAA: in addition to the negative P in V$_1$, the P's are notched in inferior leads.

130. I: NSR with sinus arrhythmia, 80/min. PR .11, QRS .08, QT normal. Normal ECG.

C: This is a nice demonstration of sinus arrhythmia, a sign of good cardiac health (see text).

131. I: ST 110/min. PR .18, QRS .08, QT normal (QTc .43). Axis −10°. Abnormal due to ST elevation in anterolateral leads; consider ischemia, but cannot exclude pericarditis. Clinical correlation needed. Small inferior Q's noted.

C: The ST's have a (normal) upwardly concave shape, and there is ST elevation in multiple vascular distributions. Pericarditis is a real possibility. Take a careful history and listen for a friction rub before committing this patient to thrombolytic therapy. Also, find an old ECG for comparison in case this is early repolarization (though it does not look like it to me—the ST's are too high).

132. I: ST 110/min. PR .20, QRS .16, QT long for the rate. Axis 120°. Abnormal due to the rhythm, RBBB + LPFB, anterior MI of uncertain age.

C: The P waves are not obvious: I believe I see them in V$_1$. This is another example of MI diagnosed in the face of RBBB. Before the anatomy of the infranodal conduction system was understood, the fascicular blocks were called peri-infarction block. Most cases of fascicular block are not caused by MI, but this may be a case of true peri-infarction block.

Perhaps the worst prognostic finding on this resting ECG is sinus tachycardia. Recall that resting tachycardia may indicate poor left ventricular function after MI. An anterior MI that injures enough of the interventricular septum to cause bifascicular block is probably a large one.

133. I: NSR 75/min. PR .16, QRS .09, QTc .60. Axis 60°. Abnormal due to long QT, T wave changes consistent with anterolateral ischemia, possibly non-Q MI.

C: The T wave changes are typical of non-Q wave infarction. Some patients with these findings do not have elevated cardiac enzymes. For this reason, I do not make the diagnosis of MI on the ECG report, but leave that to the clinician who is evaluating all the data. Q waves are different: with Q's you can make the diagnosis of MI.

This patient had an intracranial bleed, and these ECG changes are a relatively common complication of that illness. In addition to deep T inversion, marked prolongation of the QT is typical. The ECG changes come from the heart, not the head. The presumed mechanism is massive catecholamine discharge caused by the acute bleed, severe vasoconstriction, and subendocardial ischemia. Pathologic studies have shown subendocardial myolysis and an absence of coronary obstructive disease.

134. I: Sinus tachycardia, 110/min. AV sequential pacemaker with ventricular pacing.

C: This looks like LBBB. But pacer spikes are apparent in II, aVF, aVR, and V$_4$ through V$_6$.

How can you have tachycardia with a pacemaker? Is this a run-away pacer? With VVI units (single chamber, ventricular sensing and pacing), the pacer is set to fire at a fixed rate, usually 70 to 75/min. But with the DDD pacer (dual chamber, with atrial and ventricular sensing and pacing), the pacemaker will follow the atrium's lead, and sinus tachycardia with ventricular pacing is possible. There is an upper rate limit, which is usually set at 120 to 130/min.

Dual-chamber pacing is particularly good for this old person with heart failure. She is able to raise her heart rate with exercise, and atrial contraction is preserved. Loss of atrial contraction may cause cardiac output to fall 20% or more in a setting of poor LV function.

135. I: NSR 80/min. PR .18, QRS .08, QT normal. Axis 85°. Abnormal due to low QRS voltage, inferolateral ischemia, probably acute MI. Cannot exclude prior septal MI.

C: As the ST elevation involves multiple vascular distributions (inferior and lateral), could this be pericarditis? The reciprocal ST depression in aVL, V$_1$, and V$_2$ makes ischemia the likely diagnosis (reciprocal changes are not seen with pericarditis; see Table 2.4).

Should he have thrombolytic therapy? The absolute magnitude of ST elevation is not that great, suggesting this is a small MI. But there is reciprocal ST depression, a marker of larger inferior MI. ST elevation in V$_5$ and V$_6$ suggests that this man's right coronary artery supplies a portion of the lateral as well as the inferior wall. On balance, I suspect this is a large MI. At age 56, he should have reperfusion therapy.

136. I: NSR 95/min with PVC's. PR .18, QRS .10, QT long (QTc .48). Axis 20°. Abnormal due to long QT, LAA, and NSST-TCs.

C: As he was having chest pain at the time of the ECG, the ST-T changes probably are ischemic, a clinical diagnosis. You can be more certain about ischemia by comparing this with a previous ECG. ST depression that develops with chest pain indicates ischemia. He also was in pulmonary edema. After diuresis, the LAA resolved; these P wave changes may vary with left atrial pressure.

137. I: NSR 80/min. PR variable from .06 to .12, QRS variable from .06 to .10, QT normal. Axis variable. Abnormal due to intermittent pre-excitation.

C: I have mentioned that conduction across an accessory pathway may be intermittent. In this case it seems to vary with the respiratory cycle. Note the T wave changes that appear with the delta wave; it should be no surprise that changing the sequence of ventricular activation may also change the sequence of repolarization.

138. I: NSR 70/min with Mobitz I second-degree AV block (Wenckebach) and 4:3 conduction. PR variable, QRS .08, QT normal. Axis −10°. Abnormal due to rhythm, inferior MI, possibly acute.

C: If we had serial ECGs for comparison, we would call this inferior MI with evolutionary changes rather than possibly acute. There is some residual ST elevation and reciprocal ST depression, but Q's have developed. AV nodal block may persist for days or even a couple of weeks after the acute inferior infarction. The node usually recovers, either because of good collateral flow or because of relaxation of vagal tone.

139. I: ST 120/min. PR .08, QRS .08, QT normal. Axis 45°. Abnormal due to short PR, probable pre-excitation, and NSST-TCs.

C: Some patients with pre-excitation do not have a delta wave. Presumably, their bypass tract is near the AV node, so that the sequence of ventricular activation is near normal. (This is the Lown-Ganong-Levine syndrome caused by pre-excitation through the paranodal James bundle.)

140. I: NSR 80/min. PR .08, QRS .10, QT long for the rate. Axis 10°. Abnormal due to pre-excitation (WPW) and NSST-TCs. Since the prior ECG, a delta wave has developed.

C: Patients with pre-excitation may have multiple accessory pathways; this patient has switched from one to another with the change in heart rate. There has been a change in the T wave and QT interval with the change in AV conduction.

141. I: NSR 90/min. PR .18, QRS .11, QT long (QTc .52). Axis 30°. Abnormal due to biatrial abnormality, IVCD, and long QTc.

C: No comment—this seems fairly obvious at this point, right?

142. I: Multifocal atrial tachycardia 120/min. PR variable, QRS .09, QT normal. Axis 110°. Abnormal due to MAT, RAD, PRWP.

C: This much variability in the P waves and PR interval indicates either wandering atrial pacemaker (with heart rate <100; ECG No. 68) or MAT. The delay in R wave progression is consistent with her obstructive lung disease. With a deeper S wave in V_6, you could argue for RVH.

143. I: ST 110/min. PR .16, QRS .08, QT long (QTc .48). Axis 100°. Abnormal due to rhythm, acute inferolateral MI with reciprocal ST changes.

C: The ECG computer read this as possible anterior subendocardial ischemia, in addition to inferior MI. Multiple studies have tested the significance of reciprocal ST depression during inferior MI. The one thing that they agree on is that it is a marker of large infarction. Based on available evidence, I do not think reciprocal ST depression reliably points to multivessel coronary disease and ischemia in a second vascular distribution. Instead, it simply indicates that the infarct artery is a large one.

144. I: ST 120/min. PR .16, QRS .10, QT normal. Axis 90°. Abnormal due to LAA, acute anterolateral MI, and inferior MI of uncertain age.

C: This is his second MI, and it is a big one. With cardiogenic shock, the prognosis is poor unless reperfusion therapy can be accomplished quickly. For it to work, the infarct artery should be opened within 6 hours of the onset of pain. Beyond that, there is much less chance for success. Move in the direction of the cardiac catheterization laboratory as soon as you make the diagnosis of cardiogenic shock. *Do not wait to see if thrombolytic therapy will work.* If there is no catheterization laboratory in your hospital, start rT-PA therapy and call the helicopter for emergency transfer.

145. I: NSR 90/min. PR .14, QRS .09, QT normal. Axis 20°. Abnormal due to diffuse ST elevation, possibly pericarditis. Small inferior Q's noted.

C: ST elevation is seen in anterior, lateral, and inferior leads. The normal upward concavity of the ST's is maintained. Pericardial changes on the ECG are common early after heart surgery. The postcardiotomy syndrome is acute pericarditis that occurs weeks later. This patient had fever, elevation of the sedimentation rate (the key laboratory study), pleuropericardial pain, and flu-like symptoms. He responded to prednisone therapy. With these ST changes, you can see how primary care physicians or emergency room doctors might mistake it for acute infarction. But the ECG changes are typical for pericarditis.

146. I: ST 100/min, PR .16, QRS .07, QT normal. Axis 45°. Abnormal due to diffuse ST elevation, probably acute ischemia (both anterior and inferior MI).

C: The ST changes in the anterior leads look like transmural ischemia. Perhaps there is a hint of upward convexity, but I do not think so. On the other hand, the ST elevation in inferior leads is impressive, and diffuse, multiregion ST elevation suggests pericarditis. Is this simultaneous anterior and inferior infarction? Lead aVL is a teaser, as there is a hint of reciprocal ST depression (a sign of ischemia). Without clinical data, it is best to hedge when reading the ECG. If unsure at the bedside, consider emergency angiography.

147. I: Nodal tachycardia, 105/min. QRS .10, QT long (QTc .48). Axis 90°. Abnormal due to rhythm, NSST-TCs.

C: Retrograde P waves distort the T waves. Could this be a lateral MI with a Q wave in aVL?

148. *I: Probable nodal rhythm, 70/min. QRS .14, QTc .48. Axis −70°. Abnormal due to the rhythm, LAFB, IVCD, and acute anterolateral MI.*

C: I do not see P waves, although the notched ST segment in V_1 and V_2 may be the retrograde P. This looks like a huge MI; one of my colleagues refers to ST's like these as "tombstones." That is the shape, isn't it? Compared with old ECGs, the LAFB was new. There may be RBBB, hard to diagnose because of the ST changes in V_1.

149. *I: Sinus arrest with junctional escape rhythm, 32/min. QRS .10, QT normal. Axis 70°. Abnormal due to rhythm, acute inferior ischemia, probably MI.*

C: Junctional or nodal rhythm implies that the sinoatrial rate has slowed below that of the AV nodal pacemaker, and it has assumed control. In this case, the SA pacer has slowed too much, enough that I am calling it SA arrest. This patient required a temporary pacemaker.

150. *I: NSR 65/min. PR .16, QRS .08, QT normal. Axis uncertain. Probably normal ECG; suspect arm lead reversal.*

C: This is a relatively common occurrence (we staged it for this purpose with one of the technicians). A relatively young person has a bizarre axis and lateral Q waves. The axis does not fit any specific syndrome (such as RVH). Lead misplacement is the logical explanation. If you (mentally) roll lead I around its baseline, the P, QRS, and T would all be upright—the equivalent of correcting the placement of the right and left arm electrodes. Another common lead misplacement involves the V leads and bizarre R wave progression across the precordium (i.e., the R in V_3 is shorter than those in V_2 and V_4).

Index